Medical Ethics
and the
Elderly:
A Case Book

Medical Ethics and the Elderly: A Case Book

Mark H. Waymack, Ph.D.
Assistant Professor of Philosophy and
Adjunct Assistant Professor of Medical Humanities
Loyola University of Chicago

and

George A. Taler, M.D.
Assistant Professor of Family Medicine and
Director of the Division of Geriatrics
University of Maryland School of Medicine

92 91 90 89 88   5 4 3 2 1

Library of Congress Catalog Card Number: 88-60976

ISBN: 0-944496-01-6

Pluribus Press, Inc.
160 East Illinois Street
Chicago, Illinois 60611

Printed in the United States of America

Contents

Foreword

Medical ethics is an old subject and it keeps coming back anew. With his oath, Hippocrates first addressed what should be proper professional behavior in the care of patients. Ever since, generation after generation of practitioners have continued to write on this theme. In 1803, Thomas Percival, as one notable example, re-addressed the conduct of physicians and surgeons with a much longer and detailed *Medical Ethics, a Code of Institutes and Precepts,* that included advice on interprofessional behaviors. Early in this century, long before the "high tech" developments of modern medicine that can sustain life when organs fail, and when physicians feared upsetting (or losing) patients by informing them of fatal diagnoses, Richard C. Cabot wrote about medical ethics with his essay on "truth telling." The doctor must tell the truth when communicating diagnosis and prognosis. The information does not harm the patient, as physicians in the 1980s have finally recognized.

Numerous writings about the rights and duties of patients and doctors have continued to appear, both guiding and inspiring with their religious and philosophical ideas about care in society. Whether studied by the reflective practitioner, ignored by the practical-minded clinician, or read by the informed patient and consumer-interest groups of the 1980s, medical ethics texts are now constantly produced. They are almost a literary industry that seems to have developed in the wake of today's numerous medical technologies, perhaps because applications of those technical advances are now viewed as potentially hazardous even when promoted as helpful and curative in the care of the individual patient.

Yet, as Mark Waymack and George Taler, the authors of *Medical Ethics and the Elderly,* note, the rationale for modern medical ethics texts derives from more than the use of technology alone. Rather, it derives from the many changes in and out of medical practice—in the patients, organization, content and the social context of practice.

Patients today are different. As the book's title suggests, those seeking medical care are more often elderly than at any time in the past. They bring more morbid disorders for potential intervention, come with new expectations for negotiation and decision making with the staff, and hold new notions of their social and self-worth despite the frailties of their bodies and the miseries of their minds. For both patients and doctors, the organization of care is also different. More health professionals, physicians in particular, work in corporate arrangements that may constrain their traditional autonomy. Such corporate employment in turn brings third-parties into the discourse between doctor and patient, making the doctor a divided advocate of the patient. As mentioned, the content of practice today contains many more technologies. These technologies bring with them their own specialized technicians that increase the number of staff surrounding the now almost antique dyadic encounter of doctor and patient. The added staff, along with patients' families, now wants to be involved in decision making so that the negotiation between doctor and patient becomes a much larger, diverse exchange. Finally, alongside these changes in patients, organization and content of medical practice, come the political, economic and social influences of government, industry and special interest groups. These public and private payors all raise the specter, if not the reality, of limited resources for care in society. No wonder there are new questions about rights, duties and proper medical actions. Indeed, many are skeptical that the individual can be assured of personal and optimal treatment in our mass society.

Mark Waymack and George Taler's book recognizes these many changes in medical practice that again make medical ethics a new theme today. Their text focuses on specific cases—a case-oriented reader. It takes the reader through specific medical ethical problems derived from case reports of elderly patients and their caretakers. With each case the clinical and ethical actions are reviewed and ethical principles examined. A didactic text, *Medical Ethics and the Elderly* is meant to instruct, and indeed, that it does; but its teaching method is a modern inductive approach. The material goes from the clinical facts to the principles of action. As a result, it should appeal to readers of all ages. Students and young practitioners can easily follow the illustrative cases with their models of ethical reasoning; the more experienced practitioners can bring their added experiences to the reading of the cases, comparing their own thinking about what to do with the ethical discourse in the book's case reports; even lay readers can handle the text.

Readers of this volume will benefit from learning the complexities of decision making with patients and families, the principles of ethical reasoning, and the modern communication goals of doctor-patient relationships. In today's practice, learning about the patient's choices of care and treatment has a new importance alongside the traditional focus of the clinical method on getting information for accurate diagnosis. Besides eliciting complaints of bodily and emotional distress for diagnosis, medicine's discourse with patients must increasingly communicate about treatment—in effect, about the values patients hold about dying, suffering, and wanting to know (or not) their hidden risks for disease. This volume takes the reader in these important directions.

John D. Stoeckle, M.D.
Professor of Medicine, Harvard Medical School
Physician, Massachusetts General Hospital

Preface

This book results from a shared interest in bringing philosophical reflection to the pressing ethical concerns of clinical care for the elderly. Its conviction is that philosophy can gain in value by engagement with the concerns and crises of life, and medicine can benefit from the insights and thoughtfulness of philosophy.

While a visiting faculty member in philosophy at the University of Maryland Baltimore County, M.H.W. spent one morning each week with members of the Department of Family Medicine at the School of Medicine. This arrangement was mutually advantageous, since it provided an ethics forum for Family Medicine residents during their in-patient service and also provided him with hands-on experience with the reality of medical problems and practice not usually witnessed from the "ivory tower." G.A.T., Director of the Division of Geriatrics in the Department of Family Medicine at the School of Medicine, was eager to bring some ethical coherence and understanding to the care of the elderly.

This book is the product of our many discussions, arguments, disagreements, and our eventual coming to terms. It is without doubt a far better book than either of us would have written individually.

A number of people deserve thanks for their help along the way. We must begin by noting that the interest of Edward J. Kowalewski, M.D., Chairman of the Department of Family Medicine at the University of Maryland School of Medicine, laid the groundwork for our cooperation. He has also read parts of the manuscript and his comments certainly improved it. We also thank Elizabeth Kramer, John Stoeckle, M.D., and John Lynch, M.D., who patiently read various versions of the manuscript and made many valuable suggestions. Our colleagues at Loyola and the University of Maryland and our graduate students and fellows who have read and commented on various parts of the text also deserve acknowledgement. While our work has benefited from the criticisms of these people, any mistakes or errors that remain can only be our responsibility.

Finally, it has been the elderly persons in our lives who have taught us much that is in this book. G.A.T. dedicates his contributions to the memory of Paul Vernon Renoff, his father-in-law, whose death during the preparation of the manuscript made the concerns of this work a most personal and poignant experience. M.H.W. dedicates his contributions to his maternal grandmother, Gladys Johnson Fore, a victim of Alzheimer's disease who died as this manuscript was completed, and to Alena Campbell Duncan, a person who has taught him much about how to endure the challenges of personal loss and infirmity in old age with courage and spirit.

M.H.W.
Chicago, IL

G.A.T.
Baltimore, MD

March, 1988

Introduction

A good story has an appropriate ending. It may be happy or sad. If we are lucky, it is ennobling. In the story of human life, the ending frequently is old age. Concluding our lives in old age offers the opportunity for a well written story, for doing so provides the spaces for a beginning as well as for a middle period full of interesting events. Yet, even with a fine beginning and a full, interesting, and rewarding middle, the closing chapters of a story can betray our hopes. This book offers the reader, particularly the health care professional, what insights and practical suggestions we have to help the health care professional assist his or her elderly patients in their health needs as they work their way through the closing chapters of their lives, whether those closing chapters span one year or twenty.

Providing health care for the elderly raises ethical issues that we must face, as health care professionals, moral philosophers, and members of society. Though ethical issues surrounding health care for the elderly are not entirely new, they are issues which have become increasingly obvious and pressing in recent years. For one thing, a substantially increased average life span has meant that a far larger percentage of the population is reaching old age than ever before. Furthermore, advanced medical technology has made it possible to extend the lives of the ill elderly far longer than was possible in the past. While for many elderly persons, this has meant added years of vigor and fulfillment, there are also many elderly for whom this means added years of chronic suffering, dementia, and/or dependence.

One kind of ethical issue that arises in providing health care for the elderly is an allocation issue of how much and of what sort of resources should be allocated for care of the elderly. Daniel Callahan's *Setting Limits* (1987) and Norman Daniel's *Am I My Parents' Keeper* (1987) have successfully brought to public attention the ethical questions and dilemmas involved in deciding how much should be spent on health care for the elderly and who is responsible for paying for that care. These broad issues of social policy are of great importance to ourselves and our society and need our attention and voice.

A different set of ethical concerns surrounding health care for the elderly can be described as questions of *clinical ethics*. These are the day-to-day ethical questions that arise in the course of caring for particular elderly patients, elderly persons who present themselves with health care needs. Unlike issues of social policy, clinical ethics with respect to health care for the elderly has not received widespread public attention. The importance of clinical geriatric ethics has, however, attracted the efforts of several talented individuals, including Christine Cassel, Joanne Lynn, Sally Gadow, Stephen Miles, Marshall Kapp, and David Thomasma. By exploring as yet unexplored areas of geriatric ethics, by furthering discussion already begun, and by providing a sustained treatment of a broad scope of ethical issues in one volume, we hope to contribute to this important discussion.

Geriatric Ethics as a Special Topic

One might question the ethical wisdom of writing a book on medical ethics and the *elderly*. It might be objected that doing so is morally denigrating to the elderly. After all, though their bodies may change with age, the elderly are still persons deserving of moral respect just as much as when they were young or middle-aged. Pretending that there is such a thing as geriatric ethics would be, therefore, morally insulting.

We heartily agree that the elderly are just as much persons deserving moral respect as their younger counterparts. And we also agree that much of what we discuss in this book will not apply to all elderly persons, for we are focusing upon the elderly person who is a *patient*. As the reader will discover, it is not our intention to isolate the elderly or to strip them of their rights; rather it is to point out to the health care professional how many of the habits of modern medical practice unethically strip the elderly of their rights. We seek to point out how this can happen and provide suggestions on how to remedy the situation.

The Need for Clinical Geriatric Ethics

Health care professionals should not overlook the fact that the elderly present not only special physiological needs related to aging, but that there are special ethical issues which arise in the care of the elderly. While these ethical issues may not be entirely peculiar to the elderly, they are most prevalent among the elderly. They may result from societal views of the aged, expectations of the aged as compared to younger persons, value judgments concerning quality versus quantity of life, or emerging questions concerning the benefits of modern medical intervention.

An open and engaging exploration of these ethical issues is especially important for two reasons. First, there is a lack of consensus among patients, members of the medical professions, and the public at large concerning these issues. And second, there are several reasons which have made these issues more pressing in recent years than in times past. Let us first consider some of the sources of ethical disagreement and then turn our attention to the pressures which require us now to address these issues.

Sources of Ethical Disagreement or Confusion
To begin with, there is ethical disagreement among members of society at large. This is a problem which any ethically reflective person must face. It is important that the health care providers, especially physicians, recognize the diversity among value systems of their elderly patients. On occasion, and more often than we might wish to acknowledge, a patient's value system will be at odds with that of the physician or of the health care team as a whole. Physicians and other health care personnel must be sensitive to this possibility and have the ability to deal with these differences.

Second, a diversity in ethical values is reflected among practicing physicians. What one physician sees as an ethically clear cut case, another might see as fraught with ambiguity. Where one physician may see only a physiological problem requiring a straightforward solution, another physician might see an ethical quandary of great complexity. If the profession is to work in the best interests of the patient, then physicians must recognize these significant ethical differences amongst themselves and learn to resolve them.

Third, there is often ethical disagreement between the various professionals involved in the team approach to health care for the elderly. Although each of the different professions (such as medicine, nursing, and social work) has the welfare of the patient as its goal, differences in training and the nature of their relationships with elderly persons may lead them to see the welfare of the patient from their own perspectives. As the physician is generally regarded as the leader of the health care team, he or she must be able to recognize this as a source of ethical disagreement and learn how to lead the team to a workable ethical consensus.

There are further sources of ethical conflict which are more peculiar to the care of the elderly. First, there has been a revolution in the nature of modern medical care and its delivery. The role which the contemporary physician plays is quite different from the role of the practicing physician in the first quarter of this century. The revolution in medical ethics in the 1960s has done much to change medicine from a priestly or paternalistic profession into one in which patients are expected and required to exercise their own choice-making capacity. Additionally, the technological revolution in medicine has vastly increased the number of choices which a patient may be required to consider. When these two factors are combined, it is easy to understand why many older patients may have difficulty fitting comfortably into the modern medical system. This can also cause a generational difference among health care professionals themselves, arising from when they were trained in their profession.

Furthermore, even if the nature of medicine had remained static, there would remain a difference of perspective as a result of age itself. First, our society has rather negative stereotypes of the elderly. These negative attitudes can denigrate the dignity of the elderly and can have an adverse influence on the nature and quality of the health care which they receive. Second, age naturally can lead to different perspectives on life. A young intern, medical resident, or nurse may think of the possibilities that life may hold for them, the challenges of the future. Many elderly persons, however, naturally view their life as history more than as future possibilities. (Thomasma 1986) There is much of note behind them, worthy of pride and remembrance, and little in the future. Hence, what a young resident might see as a gloomy outlook on life might really be an elder person's warm satisfaction with a life well-spent and lack of morbid concern with the relatively short time left.

Pressures That Bring These Issues to the Forefront
While several of these sources of ethical disagreement or confusion may have been present for some time, there are several factors which have made these issues more pressing than ever before.

First, a variety of factors have combined to heighten cost-consciousness in health care resource allocation for the elderly. Economic incentives and constraints have been imposed upon the health care system, particularly on some of those segments which most directly affect the elderly (such as DRG regulations concerning hospital reimbursement and more narrowly defined regulations in home care and skilled institutional care). Administrators, therefore, are under pressure (not of their own choosing) to increase surveillance of utilization and expenses. They pass these pressures along to the physicians within their facilities, who now need to be sensitive to professional standards, patient preferences, and financial constraints in decisions affecting the individuals directly under their care.

Second, the emergence of the team approach to providing health care to the elderly, while offering many advantages, has altered the ethical complexion of the relationships between the members from the various professions as well as the relationship between the physician and the patient.

Third, advances in medicine have enabled physicians to diagnose and treat many diseases which previously were beyond cure or control. These developments have been successful in keeping more people alive longer and in increasing the numbers of disabled and dependent individuals. Unfortunately, our wisdom in knowing when and when not to apply such measures has not, from an ethical point of view, progressed as rapidly as the technology.

Furthermore, as a result of our success in keeping persons alive longer, there are now many elderly persons who, instead of dying quickly from some acute attack, suffer from chronic, irreversible, and degenerative diseases. As practitioners, we must, therefore, face the ethical issues raised by the care of persons with such diseases, both mental (such as dementia) and physical.

Methodology

This book seeks to avoid dependence upon an abstract, abstruse, and frequently contentious hierarchy of ethical principles. Instead, it makes use of a case-example approach to ethical discussion and analysis. At the same time, it attempts to present and discuss case examples in such a way that the reader will be able to apply these strategies in a wide variety of cases.

Towards this end, the general structure of these chapters is to begin with a case example relevant to the topic at hand. Then, the kinds of ethical values that are involved are brought to light and discussed. Finally, a portion of each chapter is devoted to an exploration of the relevant ethical issues through an analysis of the case example. All the case examples are drawn from the experience of professionals in geriatrics and gerontology.

We think this method is preferable for several reasons. First, such a presentation is particularly useful to practitioners. While academic philosophers may have the leisure to delve indefinitely into the ethical principles or values involved in these cases, medical practitioners are best served by concise discussions which may be easily applied to their everyday practice. Case-example studies are ideal for that purpose.

Second, systems of ethics which reduce our experience of the moral world into an elegant system of abstract principles are sometimes useful as heuristic devices. However, when brought to bear against real life situations rather than cleverly constructed philosophers' examples, they fail to satisfy. A case-example method, on the other hand, by using examples drawn from real experience, is more likely to constructively confront the complexity of certain morally difficult situations which face the medical professional.

Third, because the case examples are based upon real experience, they are more likely to make sense to the practicing medical professional, to grip the moral imagination of such a reader.

Finally, any endeavor in medical ethics must face the moral pluralism which characterizes this society. The most plausible approach to such divisive forces is the use of case examples conjoined with morally sensitive and helpful discussion. This is what we hope the reader will find in the following pages.

There are certain values which appear frequently in the literature of medical ethics and which are useful in defining lines of thought. A short list includes autonomy, beneficence, nonmaleficence, and justice. This book presupposes some familiarity with such terms. For those readers, however, who lack such a background, and for others who might find such a device useful as a reference, a brief glossary is located after the book's concluding chapter.

Other values are often relevant, however, and should not be casually ignored. For instance, the moral importance of personal or professional integrity, or the obligations of a physician as a spouse or parent as opposed to his or her moral obligations in a professional capacity, should not be excluded from consideration. Hence, in our case discussion, we will not restrictively limit our analysis to those specific ethical principles commonly recognized in works on medical ethics.

Divisions of the Book

This book is divided into four Parts.

Part I has the patient-provider relationship as its theme, and examines ethics and the dynamics of decision making in care for the elderly. Chapter 1 seeks to clarify the ethical responsibility of the health care professional in guiding patient care decision making. Chapter 2 examines how the patient-provider dynamics of decision making may vary in relation to the cognitive status of the patient. Chapter 3 turns to the largely unexplored area of the ethics of family involvement in decision making for elderly patients. Chapter 4 explores the challenges of decision making by the health care team as a whole. Chapter 5 explores the nature and function of institutional ethics committees and how they can be a resource for the health care professional seeking assistance in decision making. And chapter 6 points out how the possibility for participation in research poses both opportunities and challenges for the elderly patient and the care provider.

Part II tackles specific diagnostic and treatment issues made possible by the advancement of medical technology. Our theme in this part is that ethical decision making concerning diagnostic and treatment options requires that the health care provider understand the patient's perspective as an individual, including the very important fact that we are considering *elderly* patients. We have to understand how the health care goals of elderly patients may be quite different from the goals of much younger people. Quality of life, from the point of view of the elderly person, becomes an important consideration in decisions concerning medical intervention. Chapter 7 opens this part with questions, previously little discussed, concerning the ethical dimension of diagnostic interventions and the possibility of limiting such interventions for ethical reasons. Chapter 8 then considers limited treatment in general. Then there are several chapters concerning specific sorts of limitations to treatment or intervention: Chapter 9 considers the ethics of withholding or withdrawing nutrition and hydration; chapter 10 considers limits to resuscitative efforts; and chapter 11 examines the professionally sensitive issues of assisted suicide and active euthanasia for the elderly.

Part III explores the ethical dimension of the locus of care. Our thesis here is that different institutions stand for different values, goals, and needs or purposes. Thus, in discussing questions concerning the best place for delivery of health care, the health care professional must help clarify the patient's values, goals, and needs so that the patient can be matched *appropriately* with a care institution. Chapter 12 considers the hospital setting for care and what it means. Chapter 13 examines the long-term care setting and its values, goals, and needs. And chapter 14 considers the ethical implications of the home as the locus of care.

Finally, Part IV examines the role of finances in health care decision making. When is it morally proper to regard finances and reimbursement policies as ethically acceptable decision factors, and when would it be morally unacceptable to be influenced by finances?

Ethics is complex, and we cannot offer the reader magical ethical formulae or cookbook solutions to problems of clinical ethics. But by helping the reader perceive the ethical complexion of many health care decisions and by providing some ideas on how to approach these ethical issues in a constructive manner, we believe this study will be useful for all those who care for the elderly, whether or not they agree with our particular conclusions and suggestions.

Part I

Patient–Provider Relationships

CHAPTER 1

The Physician's Responsibilities in Ethical Decision Making

The Case of Dr. Simmons and Mrs. Silverthorne

"As an intern on rotation at a community hospital, I was assigned the care of Mrs. Silverthorne, who was admitted for the umpteenth time for refractory heart failure. Mrs. Silverthorne's personal doctor happened to be the attending physician on our service that month, and was a personal friend of her daughter. After bringing Mrs. Silverthorne through several episodes of pulmonary edema—the last culminating in a full cardiopulmonary arrest and resuscitation—I was taken aback when Mrs. Silverthorne asked me why I worked so hard when she was quite content to die! She bemoaned her daughter's refusal to consider a 'do-not-resuscitate' order and the fact that her physician would not honor her own decision. She begged me to help her and asked that I not discuss this further with her doctor or daughter for fear that they would somehow interfere. With mixed feelings, I promised to abide by her wishes 'the next time.'

"Several evenings later, while on night-call, I was STAT-paged to the nurse's station. Mrs. Silverthorne was in pulmonary edema, again. Despite the intravenous diuretics and morphine and oxygen, it became clear that she wasn't responding. Then she looked at me. Between gasps she exclaimed, 'You promised!' and fainted. I didn't call the emergency room attending physician who conducted the resuscitation protocols. Instead, I sat next to her on the bed and she died in my arms a few moments later.

"The nurses came to me individually to offer their support for our 'little conspiracy.' The next morning the attending physician paused for some time after I recounted the evening's events. To my surprise, he thanked me for doing 'what was right.' Even Mrs. Silverthorne's daughter wished me well, although I am not sure that she learned all the details of my care for her mother."

1.1 Introduction

This chapter brings to the foreground some aspects of what we believe is involved in establishing an ethically constructive relationship between a health care professional and his or her elderly patient. The case of Mrs. Silverthorne raises many of these issues and provides an introduction to the major themes of Part I. These are the physician's obligations to both himself and to the profession, our relationships with the patient and his or her family, and our professional relationships within the health care team. Only after laying this foundation can we address other ethically significant treatment decisions which hold particular relevance in the care of the elderly.

Although the most obvious concern would seem to be a disagreement over resuscitation status, the real issue is that of doctor-patient communication. Mrs. Silverthorne and her doctor were not alone. In a revealing article by Bedell, et al. (1983), it was pointedly shown that the vast majority of physicians avoid discussing the issues of determining CPR status with their patients. This was even true of those in the study who expressed the belief that physicians have an ethical obligation to inform patients of their medical status and to respect their patients' wishes.

Mrs. Silverthorne's doctor essentially chose to ignore her requests to refrain from CPR. This failure may come from the discomfort we all have in discussing death, a view that death is a mark of physician failure, or paternalism. In either case, the physician demonstrated a lack of preparedness for what was inevitably a not unforeseen circumstance.

The other failure in this relationship was the physician's lack of respect for the patient's autonomy. Certainly, Mrs. Silverthorne's condition could have clouded her cognitive abilities or led her to feelings of depression. However, she was able to make her wishes known most clearly to Dr. Simmons and he was able to act accordingly. The doctor-patient relationship is founded on this kind of mutual trust and interpersonal regard. The physician brings knowledge, judgment and skills; the patient then chooses among the options in accordance with his or her own values; and together a plan of diagnosis and treatment is pursued.

A second issue was the relationship that the attending physician established with the daughter. There is an unfortunate tendency when dealing with the elderly to turn to the family for decision making, as if with children. Older patients are fully competent adults, unless formally determined otherwise, and are entitled to all the rights and privileges thereof. In the eyes of the law, therefore, adults are responsible for themselves regardless of the wishes of their family or advisors. This also raises the issue of confidentiality. It is the patient who determines who else is to be included in knowledge of his or her health, or who may be consulted for direction in the event of incapacitation. Mrs. Silverthorne was able to establish a new doctor-patient relationship which allowed her to exercise her autonomy. Dr. Simmons outlined the contingencies in the event of another acute event, maintained the confidentiality of her decision and acted as her advocate within the health care system.

The third issue involves the physician's moral obligations of beneficence and non-maleficence. Efforts to extend the length of life at all costs must be mitigated by many older persons' concerns about the present and future quality of that life. We in the health care professions must be able to shift from a curative mode to one where comfort and caring predominate. In the case above, the attending physician persisted in his aggressive approach to her illness, and consequently Mrs. Silverthorne was forced to suffer through numerous painful and essentially pointless treatments and a resuscitation which she would have preferred to avoid.

Finally, this case illustrates a health care team in dysfunction. Though not often recognized as such, *other physicians* are a part of the health care team. And, in certain circumstances, it may be a moral duty of one physician to defend a patient's interests before other physicians who might thwart them. This was the case with Dr. Simmons and Mrs. Silverthorne's personal doctor. Equally important was the fact that the nurses were not included in the decision making process and only surreptitiously supported Dr. Simmons afterwards. Difficult decisions are more easily made with the assistance, knowledge and perspectives of others. In these circumstances, all members of the health care team will become involved and a general understanding greatly facilitates their participation.

Ethically Constructive Relationships

As human beings, we have several special characteristics which are morally significant. First, and perhaps of most importance, we are endowed with reason and will. That is, as persons we can make reasoned choices about what we want to do, what we would like to have done to us, and, in a broad sense, who we want to be. This capacity has come to be known as *autonomy,* based upon the Greek word for "self-rule." A second characteristic deserving mention is that as persons we are susceptible to a wide array of emotions, from happiness and pleasure to pain and suffering. These characteristics lead us to certain moral obligations as treating physicians. With respect to autonomy, we are obliged to respect, as far as possible, the choices that other persons make for themselves. And with respect to our capacity for pleasure or pain, we have the duties of beneficence and non-maleficence, i.e., the duty to promote the happiness and relieve the suffering of other persons, and the duty to do no harm.

Physicians, therefore, must strive to know a great deal more about their patients as persons, about their values relative to life versus disabilities and the extent to which they will accede to diagnostic and therapeutic interventions in the preservation of life. This kind of information, under ordinary circumstances, is most reliable when obtained directly from the patient, for it is the patient who is usually the best judge and most authoritative voice of what constitutes his or her abiding interests.

Obstacles to Ethically Constructive Relationships

Unfortunately, there are numerous obstacles to free and informative communication. The first may be the physician's reluctance to broach discussion. Doing so often requires that physicians share their own perceptions and philosophy with the patient. Denial of mortality is probably as common among physicians as in the general population. Death as an inevitable reality is an unsettling topic in the abstract, let alone the specifics of one's own demise. Not only is this a difficult topic to address, but a poorly handled discussion of such matters can alienate the patient: fundamental differences over the management of unanticipated problems may undermine an otherwise working relationship, or be construed as a morbid fatalism.

Patients who are now elderly grew up in a social age when the medical profession was very paternalistic, assuming the responsibilities of decision making as justified by the weight of their superior knowledge and under the rubric of beneficence and nonmaleficence. Patients were discouraged from being inquisitive or from trying to play an active role in choosing treatment plans. Hence, many elderly patients are by habituation reluctant to question a medical professional and to speak of their own wishes. Many physicians have neither the time, patience, nor inclination to cultivate a sense of mutuality.

Another reason is the prevalent, though unjustified, stereotype of elderly persons as having poor judgment. Though medical professionals may know this stereotype is false in a scientific sense, they may still be unconsciously guided by it in practice. Physicians more frequently turn to children of the elderly patient for directions on treatment choices, or may paternalistically decide on a treatment plan themselves without consulting either the patient or family. Drs. Bedell and Delbanco found that less than 20 percent of the patients resuscitated at their university teaching hospital had discussed CPR with either the attending physician or the house staff, while 33 percent of the families had been consulted. And, of the patients who survived and remained competent, there was only a weak correlation between the patient's desires and their physician's opinions about their attitudes.

It is often difficult for physicians to acknowledge the limits of the medical profession. We are trained, rewarded and revered for our promotion of health through medical and surgical cures. Many believe that an air of optimism in the face of death is an important ingredient in the curative process. To discuss abridgements or withholding of therapeutic options can undermine this vital force.

Suggested Strategies on Opening Discussion

There are quite a few strategies which might be helpful in developing a physician-patient relationship which is open to ethical discussions. First, however, the physician should develop a plan for the management of a serious illness in his or her own family. The delineation of responsible parties, completion of advance directives—including organ donation—and estate and insurance planning are helpful experiences for those who expect to counsel others.

Second, one ought to assess the patient's competency to make decisions concerning medical care. This assessment must include an emotional as well as cognitive evaluation. If the assessment reveals a significant cognitive impairment which is irreversible, then the physician is obligated to initiate the process for identifying the proper individual to assume responsibility. Emotional impairments, either personality, functional or affective disorders, may require initiating psychiatric consultation and treatment. If the patient is judged to be a reliable reporter of his or her ethical values, then it is incumbent upon the physician to foster a relationship which provides the patient with relevant information and encourages the patient to discuss his or her beliefs and wishes. (The topic of competency is discussed more fully in chapter 2.)

Third, we must become aware of our peer generation bias. Our perspectives on life are in large measure determined by our age, accomplishments, position, and family and peer relationships. These obviously change over time. Under most practice circumstances differences in personal outlook are not burdensome problems. However, in the care of the elderly, these intergenerational issues are nearly always present. The competencies, wisdom of experience and views from a different vantage in life that are held by our elderly patients must be consciously acknowledged.

One of the most profound differences among generations is one's attitude towards dying and death. The elderly are more apt to have these concerns on their minds since it is highly likely that they have encountered such situations through the experiences of close friends of their generation, their parents or spouses. By virtue of their age, older people begin to expect some untoward medical event and are coming to grips with their own mortality. There comes a time when quality of life becomes more important than quantity. This can best be handled if the physician knows the patient's considered preferences beforehand. The difficulty is in choosing the right circumstances for this discussion, when both the patient and the physician are adequately prepared.

We have found that the optimal time to broach these issues is as part of the regular annual examination. An examination of values fits comfortably with a general review of systems, social history and reevaluation of the problem list and medical regimen. Included should be Living Wills, durable power of attorney, legal wills, insurance coverage (including disability and life insurance), and post-retirement financial planning. By bringing these issues up for discussion on an annual basis, they can be discussed in a non-threatening atmosphere. Furthermore, by discussing them each year, ethical decisions can be reassessed for reaffirmation or change.

Other important benefits to the physician-patient relationship accrue through these discussions. Interpersonal bonds are solidified; the patient's judgment and reasoning capabilities are confirmed; and, there is an opportunity to cultivate a mutuality of decision making. We are far more inclined, then, to promote autonomy in the face of illness. We become far better advocates in inter-generational conflicts of opinion.

For a less formal presentation of these issues, Living Will documents can be made available along with other health education pamphlets in the waiting areas. We also use "advance packets" for introducing new patients to our practice and gathering information not always readily available (or time consuming to obtain) prior to our initial history and physical examination. This approach allows the patient the choice of timing these discussions; accompanying literature can often be obtained through the Institutional Ethics Committee, State Legislature or the Society for the Right to Die.*

Permutations

In the case of Mrs. Silverthorne, it is clear that the regular family doctor's lack of a constructive relationship with the patient led to a variety of ethically awkward situations. It is also easy to see how the situation could have been more complicated than it was.

What should the intern have done if Mrs. Silverthorne had

*Write c/o Society for the Right to Die, 250 West 57th Street, New York, New York 10107. (212) 246-6973.

been unable to reconfirm her wish not to be resuscitated? We believe that he should still have refrained from resuscitation, in concert with the patient's last wishes. However, if Mrs. Silverthorne, at the moment of crisis, indicated that she now wanted to be resuscitated, the physician should accept her apparent change of mind as indicative of Mrs. Silverthorne's true wishes.

Finally, recall that it was unclear that Mrs. Silverthorne's daughter ever knew of the events surrounding her mother's death. Health care professionals have no obligations to inform family members, such as the daughter, of the conditions and treatment choices of competent patients, although it is far preferable, with the patient's permission. However, had the daughter been present at the time of the acute exacerbation, she should be given emotional support and told that this is what the patient, herself, had requested. It would also have been helpful to share with the daughter the futility of the resuscitation efforts in these circumstances, the pain and loss of dignity involved in the procedure—which you would rather she not see—and that it is more important that she be with her mother at the time of death as a united family.

Conclusion

If we are to provide health care which respects our patients' wishes as reflected in their own values, we must make efforts to open and maintain channels of communication. This is best done by cultivating a relationship which fosters a mutuality of decision making.

1.2 The Responsibility to Broach Ethical Issues in Crisis

Many treatment decisions have to be made quickly and under circumstances which do not allow conferring with the patient. Wherever possible, it is important that the health care professional broach certain critical issues with the patient before they actually arise. The case of Dr. Buell and Mr. Campbell further illustrates this point.

The Case of Dr. Buell and Mr. Campbell

"I was asked to make house calls on Mr. Campbell since he refused to leave his home after having been beaten during a break-in and robbery. It was reported that he no longer went to bed and had tremendously swollen feet. Much to my surprise, Mr. Campbell was cognitively intact, but understandably fearful of his environment. He readily accepted an invitation to move in with a neighbor and her family. His only 'blood family' was a nephew who lived out-of-state. The nephew had assumed responsibility for his financial affairs through a power of attorney, but visited only once or twice a year.

"Mr. Campbell's physical problems quickly came under control. He blossomed, enjoying his new role as a 'grandpa.'

"Sometime later, when he developed rectal bleeding, his 'adopted' family called an ambulance which took him to the hospital. He refused all invasive procedures, but allowed transfusions which stabilized his condition until the bleeding stopped. After his discharge, he told me that he would rather die than return. We discussed the matter and I acknowledged his wishes.

"Nearly two years passed uneventfully, but then, Mr. Campbell became acutely ill with fever and obtundation. I spoke with the caregiver over the telephone. His history and symptoms pointed to urosepsis. The caregiver was uncomfortable with the prospect of Mr. Campbell dying in her home because of the closeness he had developed with her two small children. I reluctantly made arrangements for an ambulance and informed the emergency room staff that Mr. Campbell was 'no CPR, but IV's and antibiotics were appropriate.'

"The medical admitting officer decided to obtain a culture of his cerebrospinal fluid on the basis of fever and change of mental status. In the midst of the procedure, Mr. Campbell suffered a respiratory arrest and failed to respond to simple measures. The physician attempting the lumbar puncture opted for intubation and ventilatory assist. Hospital policy dictates that patients in the ICU must be managed by the critical care team. Although Mr. Campbell was alert and obviously frightened, his ability to communicate was seriously impaired and unreliable; I left a note stating Mr. Campbell's prior wishes. The nephew was called, but he felt that he was in no position to authorize the hospital to 'pull the plug.' The following day they attempted to wean him from the respirator, but after several minutes he experienced a full cardiopulmonary arrest. Because he had been previously resuscitated, a second attempt was initiated but was only partially successful. Mr. Campbell was now in a full coma, with failing systemic perfusion and impending renal failure.

"Mr. Campbell lingered on the ventilator for several more weeks. The Nephrology Service consulted but denied him dialysis and he died in renal failure shortly thereafter, having never regained consciousness."

Case Discussion

Unlike the case of Mrs. Silverthorne, Mr. Campbell's interests were not best served in the end. Despite his advanced years and infirmities, he had not clarified his wishes with his family, which left him without an advocate. Dr. Buell had a moral responsibility to remonstrate with the "family" to uphold what they previously agreed to, but could not override their decision. In this case, the "family's" wishes carry greater weight than the wishes of the "guest." A planned, in-home death must be agreed upon by the survivors and caregivers as the rights of the individual are superceded following his or her demise. (See chapters on family and home care.)

The next major issue is the decision to resuscitate following the lumbar puncture despite a verbal "no CPR" order made by the referring physician. We believe that the decision was fundamentally correct. A patient's wish to refrain from CPR is usually based upon the vision of end-stage, irreversible disease; death results from a natural progression of decline. What the medical admitting officer faced, however, was not someone dying "naturally," but someone who had arrested as a consequence of a medical intervention. In this instance, the physician was actively involved in a procedure which has a known morbidity and mortality rate. This active role at the time of cardiac arrest implies a degree of complicity and a sense of unnecessary death, both of which should be righted. Furthermore, the physician is acting as a professional employed by the hospital, and hospital policy usually dictates that CPR be initiated in such cases of unforeseen arrest. It is ethically understandable, therefore, that in such a crisis situation the emergency physician chose in favor of trying to preserve a life.

The picture changes, however, as it becomes clear that Mr. Campbell is suffering from an irreversible condition. Dr. Buell acted properly by letting the critical care team know about Mr. Campbell's wishes. The Nephrology Service acted in concert with these wishes in the absence of the responsible relative's decision. As his condition deteriorated, no further steps were taken to reverse the natural course.

Permutations

The major question concerns the role of the nephew. Had he agreed to the "no CPR" order, should the ICU staff have resuscitated Mr. Campbell following his second arrest? We believe so. The factors which were operant during his first arrest still held and the second resuscitation should be construed as an extension of the first. However, once his condition stabilized and the progression of his illness became more clearly defined, his wishes as conveyed through Dr. Buell were respected. Only had Mr. Campbell regained competence and refused CPR should the second attempt not have been offered.

Conclusion

Physicians are faced with both anticipated and unanticipated acute events. Care must be taken to understand the approaches appropriate to both circumstances. Where family plays a role, it is important that they be included in decisions of care in the event of acute, unforeseen illness.

1.3 The Responsibility to Confer with the Patient Concerning Current Treatment Decisions

In most instances of chronic disease, the illness has a natural and foreseeable course. The physician has the responsibility for explaining the likely course of events, the various medical options, and eliciting the patient's views on the various diagnostic and treatment interventions. When the possibility of an acute exacerbation is likely, e.g., with congestive heart failure, chronic obstructive pulmonary disease, degenerative neurological conditions, cancer, etc., anticipatory guidance from the patient deserves special consideration.

In practical terms, this discussion should take place at an annual examination, at the time of a major change in therapeutic approach, and when the need for hospitalization arises. Included should be:

(1) the appropriateness of second opinions
(2) treatment options if competence is lost
(3) the execution of a living will, or preferably, of a durable power of attorney
(4) CPR status
(5) long term ventilatory support
(6) the extent of insurance coverage or other financial matters related to such possibilities as institutionalization or chronic hospitalization.

Assuring the opportunity for these discussions is somewhat reflected in practice style as it relates to the use of acute care services. Early admission for stabilization and therapeutic "fine-tuning" before decompensation becomes critical and more often provides the situations when these decisions are both practical and appropriate. Later, in the natural course of illness, the needs for hospitalization are also in better perspective if death appears imminent (see chapter 12). Even though the discussion of these issues may cause some emotional discomfort or anxiety in both the patient and physician, it is necessary to broach them prophylactically if the moral autonomy as well as the well-being of the patient is to be preserved throughout the remainder of his or her life.

It is also important that patients be kept informed and involved in decisions concerning current treatment. The principle ethical value involved here is the autonomy of the individual. In this connection there are four topics deserving consideration.

Maintaining Professional Knowledge
The way in which a specific illness affects an individual varies with age. If physicians are to provide proper care for the elderly patient, it is necessary to maintain a degree of familiarity with the principles of geriatric medicine as well as current developments in the disease process at hand.

A Willingness to Explain That Knowledge
Patient autonomy is preserved and promoted by maintaining a working partnership and not allowing choices to be made out of ignorance. Health care professionals have a moral obligation, therefore, to take the time and effort to explain to elderly patients, in terms that they can understand, the nature of their medical conditions, therapeutic options and prognoses.

Sharing Opinions
Health care professionals should make an effort to provide a balanced view of the various options, but should be willing to state what course of action appears most preferable and explain why this is so.

Sharing the Limits of Professional Competency
Health care professionals should be forthright with their patients concerning the limits of their professional expertise. This can be seen in two contexts. First, they must be willing to admit when they are unable to make an accurate prognosis. That is, there are times when medical ignorance makes it impossible to interpret diagnostic information or to predict the future course of events. Second, physicians must be willing to inform their patients when a problem is beyond their professional expertise, and should initiate and assist in the referral to another physician with special training and experience.

(For a more complete discussion of autonomy and competency, see chapter 2.)

1.4 The Physician as Patient Advocate

The expansion and integration of service settings has created a health care *system* which has altered the physician-patient relationship in modern medicine. Hence, this relationship is no longer the dyad of "traditional" medicine, but is a triad of patient-physician-system. Part IV of this book focuses more fully upon this aspect, but the more general issue is that it is the physician's responsibility to act as advocate for his or her patient when the mechanisms of the system unjustly threaten to compromise the patient's care or choices.

The Case of Dr. Harris and Mr. Hayes

"I cared for Mrs. Hayes through her cerebrovascular disease with disabling hemiparesis, and the metastatic carcinoma which eventually took her life. During this time, I came to know Mr. Hayes, who was instrumental in defining the terms of his wife's care.

"Our interactions were both of a counselling nature in reference to his wife's illness and of a therapeutic nature in dealing with his alcoholism and heavy smoking. Shortly after his wife's death, he brought these conditions under control and we saw each other only in passing.

"The following year, Mr. Hayes came to my office having been told that he had developed inoperable cancer of the bladder. He felt that his physician was not pursuing an aggressive course with his illness, and asked for help in arranging a second opinion. On the other hand, should his condition be hopeless, he wanted me to care for him in the same way that I had cared for his wife. He then gave me a copy of his Living Will for my records and requested that he be consulted as long as he could participate in decision making, and that I withhold no information. The second surgeon was more aggressive. A pelvic exenteration removed the tumor with clear margins, and an ilial-diversion was an acceptable price to pay for several more full years.

"Three years later, he presented with nausea, hepatomegaly and weight loss. A liver biopsy revealed metastatic transitional cell carcinoma. An experimental chemotherapy protocol was offered, which Mr. Hayes declined; instead, he sought admission to the hospice service. He requested that should he become no longer able to communicate, I should do nothing to prolong his existence. He was given oral opiates for pain and when he eventually slipped into a coma, no further measures were taken. He expired the following day without the use of IV's or nasogastric tubes."

Case Discussion

Because of an open relationship with a physician who was willing to elicit, acknowledge, and accept his views, Mr. Hayes received the kind of care which he desired throughout his illness. When he desired aggressive treatment, for example, Dr. Harris assisted in finding a second surgeon willing to aggressively treat this elderly patient. When, however, Mr. Hayes decided that there was little more that he wanted done, Dr. Harris assisted in arranging hospice care in conformity with Mr. Hayes' wishes. In this case Dr. Harris' relationship with Mr. Hayes was helpful in furthering his patient's personal wishes although he was usually only peripherally involved in delivering care.

Conclusion
The health care professional must be willing to take on the role of patient advocate before the system, though there will be limits as to what can or should be done. This is true not only of the acute care institution, but also of the nursing home setting and in the patient's home.

1.5 The Physician as Leader of the Health Care Team

The ethical relationships created by the team approach to health care are the focus of chapter 4, but it is appropriate to point out here that it is the moral responsibility of the physician to accept the role of ethical leader of the health care team. This responsibility can involve various tasks.

There is a responsibility to communicate with members of the team so that others are clearly aware of their particular duties and understand the context of those duties. For example, a patient's desire not to be resuscitated can be sidetracked if other members of the team, such as nurses, are not aware that the patient has made this choice in consultation with the physician. Furthermore, not discussing such issues with the other members of the health care team can lead to alienation of some of its members, thus reducing the effectiveness of patient care.

The physician is responsible for arbitrating amongst members of the health care team when ethical conflicts arise. Although the doctor shares responsibility with the team as a whole for what is decided, society holds the physician accountable legally and financially.

The physician must also share, when appropriate, relevant information with other members of the team. There is a certain degree of physician-patient confidentiality which should be maintained, yet in doing so one could easily lead to a violation of the patient's express wishes when other team members are not aware. This issue is discussed in the next section.

1.6 Establishing the Domain of Confidentiality

Since the health care of the elderly is often provided through a team approach, questions will arise concerning the domain of physician-patient confidentiality. Consider the case of Mr. Abrams.

The Case of Dr. Turner and Mr. Abrams

"Mr. Abrams is a smallish man of 79 years, trim and attractive. His olive complexion gives him the look of a perpetual tan, neatly offset by his light gray hair. The years have been good to him physically, but as an aging homosexual his social circle has dwindled. He sees one younger man of 67 years who visits for a few hours twice a week as his sole source of companionship. Consequently, he suffers a great deal of loneliness.

"As a member of a generation which did not easily accept homosexuality, Mr. Abrams has been depressed most of his life. Though he has been frank with Dr. Turner, he has never 'announced' his homosexuality, and prefers that others not be told. Acquaintances see the sadness in his eyes and tend to shy away. He cries easily and dwells on unpleasant things, but when engaged, responds with an unexpected warmth that comes from being too long alone.

"Mr. Abrams' niece is both touched by his loneliness and buoyed by his friendship. Being widowed and living alone herself, she would be more than happy to share expenses and company by sharing households. The arrangement is appealing to Mr. Abrams, both financially and because of the social contact. But he is very concerned about the effect this would have upon his 'relationship.' The niece sees only the benefits of shared living arrangements and misconstrues his hesitancy as a reluctance to impinge upon her life. She has contacted both the office nurse of Dr. Turner's practice and the local social worker. Mr. Abrams is beginning to feel the subtle pressures whenever he visits the office."

Discussion

Traditionally, the physician-patient relationship has a strong element of confidentiality. Care for the elderly patient, however, often raises challenges to this tradition.

First, as we have frequently pointed out, the nature of health-related problems of elderly patients has made the "team" approach to health care extremely useful. Physicians, nurses, and social workers, working together, can provide far better care for the elderly patient than when they work as discrete individuals. What makes this team approach successful is that the different professional skills of the various members can be closely coordinated. But that coordination requires the sharing of pertinent information, some of which may be of a very personal nature.

The care of Mr. Abrams is a case in point. Mr. Abrams wishes to keep his secret and has divulged this information to Dr. Turner only as necessary for proper medical care. By not knowing that Mr. Abrams is hesitant to move in with his niece because of his homosexuality, the social worker (and the nurse) are pressuring Mr. Abrams to accept what they can only see as a perfectly reasonable arrangement. They cannot understand his reluctance. Yet Dr. Turner is hesitant to explain to them his reasons, since to do so would involve a breach of confidence.

Since sharing pertinent patient information with other members of the health care team can be to the patient's benefit, physicians should make an effort at the beginning of the relationship with the elderly patient to establish the domain of confidentiality. Time should be spent explaining the nature and rationale since the team approach may be unfamiliar to elderly patients. Then the patient can make an informed agreement with the physician concerning what sorts of information can be shared with what sorts of persons on the health care team without violating any personal trust.

In the case of Mr. Abrams, therefore, the physician would be well advised to approach Mr. Abrams and openly discuss his reasons for wishing to disclose the fact of his homosexuality to the social worker. For it would be to Mr. Abrams' benefit for the social worker to understand the source of tension in his relationship with his niece. It is also conceivable that the counseling skills of the social worker, with the cooperation of Mr. Abrams, could lead to a happy resolution of the matter for all involved. A responsible part of Dr. Turner's care for Mr. Abrams could, therefore, be a discussion with him of how extending the domain of confidentiality could prove beneficial to him and seeking his permission to share the relevant information.

A second way in which care for the elderly is liable to deviate from the traditional norm of physician-patient confidentiality is with respect to the family. Chapter 3 specifically addresses the ethically complex nature of the role of the family in health care for the elderly patient.

Conclusion

At least in the case of competent elderly patients, the physician can best respect the autonomy of the elderly person by discussing these issues beforehand. There should be a mutually agreeable understanding of what information can and cannot be shared with other members of the health care team or with family members without violating the confidentiality of the physician-patient relationship. It is also important for the physician to view this confidence in a larger context, for in some instances, sharing may enhance caring by removing emotional barriers. Counseling which helps the patient broaden the scope of trust to include potential caregivers can be highly beneficial.

1.7 Conclusions

We have argued in this chapter that health care professionals, and in particular physicians, are responsible for the promotion and preservation of the well-being of their patients in a manner respecting their autonomy. This requires that professionals assume a far more interactive role in ethical decision making than has often been the case. It is imperative that the patient's thoughts, beliefs, and choices concerning his or her health care be elicited rather than trusting to the opinions of family members or the health care staff itself.

This is a continual process. It involves discussion of current medical difficulties, but it also includes discussion with the patient of issues which may still only be potential difficulties. These discussions concerning ethically laden choices should not be restricted to times of severe illness, but should ideally be a part of chronic care management, and even "well patient" care.

We have also argued that the nature of modern health care for elderly persons differs in ethically important respects from the traditional image of the physician-patient relationship. Health care is usually delivered through a team approach, drawing upon the professional skills of a variety of disciplines. Furthermore, the frequency of multiple health and social problems and the highly technological and expensive nature of modern health care means that such care is now provided within an organized system of health care. These factors extend the range of the professional interaction to include the physician-patient-system relationship. Health care professionals, therefore, must understand that defending the interests of their patients within this organization is also part of their moral duties.

References

Bedell SE, and Delbanco TL. "Choices About Cardiopulmonary Resuscitation in the Hospital: When do physicians talk with patients?" *New England Journal of Medicine* 310:1089–92 (1984).

CHAPTER 2

The Patient

Modern medical ethics has emphasized the value of patient autonomy. While we are not inclined to agree that promoting patient autonomy always takes precedence, it certainly must rank as a value of very great importance. Hence, despite the prevalent stereotypes which encourage treating the elderly patient in a paternalistic fashion, the health care professional's relationship with the elderly patient, when that patient is competent, should be structured around a deep concern for patient autonomy.

Unfortunately, not all elderly patients are able to exercise autonomy. There is no doubt that the general negative social view of the aged as "needing looking after" is a gross exaggeration. Nevertheless, lack of competency is a significant problem among the elderly. Of those persons around 65 years of age, approximately 5 percent suffer from a significant mental impairment of the Alzheimer's type. At 75 years of age, that percentage increases to 7 percent. By 80 years, it grows to 10 percent. And at 85 years of age, approximately 20 percent suffer from Alzheimer's type mental impairment. (Katzman, et al., 1978) As the numbers of the old-old grow, this will become an even more prevalent problem for the health care professional.

The health care professional must therefore appeal to some ethical framework for caring for the elderly patient who can no longer exercise autonomy. The values here necessarily will be different from those which are preeminent in caring for the competent patient.

To complicate matters further, the presentation of dementia in the elderly is most often as a gradual process. Alzheimer's type dementia as well as multi-infarct dementia, both common causes of loss of mental function among the elderly, develop over a number of years. This means that there is a substantial period of time during which it would be misleading to say the patient is either truly competent or incompetent. Instead, a more accurate way of speaking is to say that there is a range of *marginal* competency which these patients occupy.

The health care professional's relationship with such patients will have a different ethical complexion than that with either the fully competent or incompetent. Some balance must be sought between (1) respecting the autonomy that remains and (2) paternalistically protecting the patient from truly undesirable harm.

Finally, we think it important to recognize non-adherence and non-compliance in elderly patients. The health care professional must be able to recognize the distinction and to see that different strategies are ethically appropriate for the different patterns of behavior.

This chapter, therefore, considers the health care professional's relationship to patients in each of these four categories: (A) the competent elderly, (B) the incompetent, (C) the marginally competent, and (D) the non-adherent and non-compliant. We argue that respecting autonomy should be strongly emphasized with regard to care for competent elderly persons. On the other hand, paternalistically protecting the welfare of the patient is the ethically correct emphasis when caring for the cognitively incompetent elderly. The more troubling category, however, is the marginally competent patients. There we advocate an ethically sensitive balancing act between preserving autonomy and protecting the patient. Finally, distinguishing between non-adherence and non-compliance, we suggest some appropriate strategies for dealing with each type of behavior.

A. The Competent Patient

The Case of Dr. Dover and Mrs. Schaefer

"As a third year resident, I took care of Mrs. Schaefer in the Health Center. She was my patient and I saw her about every three months for almost two years. Despite her troubles, she did very well for an 83-year-old. Her hus-

band had died some years before, but she had a good relationship with her son and daughter. Her diabetes and
hypertension were easily controlled. She managed her colostomy without any help. Her surgery for bowel cancer
had been over ten years ago, and as far as I was concerned
she was one of those lucky few who were actually cured.

"Mrs. Schaefer did tell me that when her time came I
should let her go. But she had never refused treatment before. In fact, she had been in just a couple of months ago
with cellulitis in her leg which she let us treat with IV antibiotics. So I assumed she would always want treatment.

"One or two days before she came in this last time,
she had dark stools which finally became frank melena.
By the time she showed up in the emergency room, her
hematocrit was in the 20's. I ordered two pints of whole
blood. She accepted the transfusions, but reluctantly. The
bleeding stopped, but just for safety's sake, we admitted
her for overnight observation.

"During the night she began to bleed again, but much
more profusely. With difficulty, I got her consent to do a
colonoscopy. Unfortunately, the colonoscopy did not re-
veal the bleeder.

"The G.I. fellow recommended angiography and oc-
clusion of the artery, but she absolutely refused any kind
of surgery. She said that her previous surgery was so awful
that she never wanted to undergo that kind of suffering
again. The fellow, the surgeon, and I all pushed her hard. I
told her that without the surgery she would most probably die. But she was adamant. I appealed to her son and
daughter, but they both said that whatever their mother
wanted was what should be done—that it was for her to
decide. Frantically, I called the attending physician and
told him the story. I was stunned when he said that I
should abide by her wishes.

"We had been pumping in transfusions through two
IV's as fast as we could, but she was bleeding even faster.
For some reason we decided that eight units would be as
far as we would go. She did not stop bleeding. All we
could do was plug her colostomy and clean her up.

"She didn't say too much. She lay there with her two

children sitting at her bedside. We all watched. The life just slowly drained from her face. Soon, she was dead."

Discussion

One very important aspect of us as persons is our capacity to make reasoned choices. We can choose what we want to do, what we do or do not want done to us, and even what kind of persons we want to be. Furthermore, it is this capacity to make reasoned choices, rather than to be simply led by blind instinct, that allows us to make sense of ourselves as beings who can be held responsible for our behavior and, hence, moral beings. Different moral theories offer different explanations of this capacity and how it fits into morality.

Immanuel Kant, eighteenth century German philosopher, called this capacity for reasoned choice "autonomy," i.e., "self-rule." Since it is our capacity for autonomy which distinguishes us from the other animals (who do not bear moral responsibilities), it is therefore this rational will which merits our citizenship in a community of moral beings. Therefore, Kant concludes, to treat another person as a *person* requires that we respect their autonomy.

John Stuart Mill, an English philosopher and economist of the nineteenth century, was a proponent of the moral theory called Utilitarianism. This theory argued that that action is morally correct which produces the greatest happiness for the greatest number of people. Mill passionately argued that one of the things which gives us the most happiness (and which causes the greatest suffering when we are deprived of it) is the ability to be in control of our own lives. To frustrate someone's liberty, therefore, detracts enormously from their happiness and is hence a morally wrong thing to do.

Aristotle also emphasized our human capacity for reasoned choice. He thought that we are most virtuous when we are actualizing our special potentials or capacities. Since our most special capacity as humans is the ability to rule our life by reasoned judgment, we are most morally admirable when we are exercising reasoned choice over the course of our lives. Thus, to ignore other persons' autonomy is to rob them of the possibility of living up to their potential as virtuous moral persons.

There are, therefore, different accounts of why the capacity for autonomy is morally important. But though the philosophical accounts given may vary, it remains true that moral theories that gain respect and credence emphasize this human capacity for autonomy.

The moral importance of our duty to respect a person's autonomy is reflected in our society's emphasis upon informed consent. If one does not obtain informed consent, then one is doing something to the other person to which he or she has not agreed. Not to obtain informed consent is not to respect the other person's capacity to make reasoned choices, and therefore fails to respect the other as a moral agent. Indeed, we value our autonomy so highly that we use the legal terms of assault and battery to describe and defend against such coercive behavior. To do an invasive procedure against a patient's wishes is to commit an illegal assault upon that person.

There are, we must hasten to add, moral and legal limitations to the exercise of autonomy. We need not always respect another person's autonomy when doing so seriously harms an innocent third party. For example, physicians are required to report the incidence of such diseases as syphilis in the interests of public health. We need not, and should not, comply with a patient's wishes if doing so would cause injustice against others. For example, we should not keep a patient in the ICU if doing so is medically unnecessary, even if he wants to stay. To do so could well prevent a truly critically ill person from finding an available ICU bed, not to mention the overuse of funds leading to unnecessarily higher health care premiums for other persons. And we need not comply with a patient's wishes when doing so would be medically inappropriate and contrary to professional standards of care.

The case of Dr. Dover and Mrs. Schaefer illustrates the tensions that can arise when a health care professional and patient have very different ideas of what ought to be done. In the case of Mrs. Schaefer's gastrointestinal bleeding, Dr. Dover's medical training, like that of most physicians, has been geared toward saving and preserving life. There was no question in her mind but that Mrs. Schaefer should undergo surgery to locate the site of the bleed and resolve the problem. She was quite taken aback, then, when Mrs. Schaefer refused permission for surgery on the grounds that she had been operated on ten years ago and never wanted to undergo that sort of torture and personal invasion again. She presumed that Mrs. Schaefer did not understand the full meaning of her refusal, and this is why she explained once again that if the surgery was not performed Mrs. Schaefer would die from a loss of blood. Nevertheless, Mrs. Schaefer remained adamant in refusal. After questioning the patient, Dr. Dover saw no reason to consider Mrs. Schaefer incompetent. The patient could give some reasons for why she did not want the surgery, though Dr. Dover thought they were not good reasons.

We believe that Dr. Dover acted properly by accepting Mrs. Schaefer's wishes, even though she thought that Mrs. Schaefer was making the wrong choice. For by accepting Mrs. Schaefer's choice, Dr. Dover was respecting her patient as a person. Differences in perspective can make it difficult to appreciate the motivation for someone else's choices. In this case, an age difference as well as professional training made it difficult for Dr. Dover to understand Mrs. Schaefer's choice. But respecting a patient's autonomy means respecting it even when one disagrees with the choice made.

This view is widely shared by medical ethicists. The President's Commission endorses the right of the competent patient to refuse treatment, even when that treatment is life saving. Nor, as some authors have specifically pointed out, should wishes of the family be able to override the wishes of the competent patient. (Younger and Jackson [1980] and Ruddick [1980].) Each of these authors argues that, even when it is life-maintaining treatment that is at issue, the autonomous wishes of the patient should be respected.

Once again, one must be careful to assess the patient's mental status. The physician in charge must make sure that the patient is saying what he or she really wants. If the physician believes that the patient is speaking under a pathological depression, then the health care professional must seriously question the competency of the patient. Similarly, a patient's expressed judgment can be regrettably influenced by a desire to exert some control over his or her own destiny in a situation where very little is left to the patient's choice. In such cases, the strong desire to exert control for the sake of exerting control can lead the patient to demand things which he or she really does not want. (As Younger and Jackson point out, this can easily occur with the machine-monitored and machine-dependent patient in a critical care unit.) Finally, physicians must be careful not to "read into" the patient's words what they want to hear, rather than what the patient is trying to say under stressful conditions.

The health care professional, therefore, has a very strong duty to respect the autonomy of elderly persons. If a situation arises where the health care professional strongly disagrees with a patient's choice, or where the choice is a particularly momentous one, involving matters of life or death, steps should be taken before acting to ensure that the patient is acting competently and expressing a sincere wish. If the health care provider is convinced that the patient is speaking competently and sincerely, then there is a moral obligation to accede to the patient's decision, even if the health care professional strongly disagrees. Alternately, as discussed in chapter 1, the health care professional may choose (under certain circumstances) to withdraw from the case, transferring the patient to someone else's care. If, however, it is felt that the patient's competency is compromised, then the ethical obligation to respect autonomy is obviated and different values come to the forefront. (Dealing with the incompetent patient is discussed in the following section of this chapter.)

We do not mean to ignore the difficulty Dr. Dover had in making her decision. As we have mentioned, health care professionals are trained to save and preserve life. This can lead us to the mistaken conclusion that preserving life is the only goal of medicine. Such a belief will frequently dictate courses of action contrary to the settled wishes of competent patients. Rather, we must be more willing to acknowledge that the goal of medicine is to serve the *overall* interests of the patient. These interests are not only the prolongation of life. As Eric Cassell has compellingly argued (1982), it is better to understand medicine as aiming to relieve suffering than simply to prolong life.

A.1 Five Common Ways in Which the Autonomy of the Elderly Is Frustrated

Unlike the case of Mrs. Schaefer, the autonomy of patients is often not respected. This is particularly true with respect to the care of the elderly. There are several ways in which the autonomy of the elderly person is peculiarly vulnerable. The first two ways are internal to the health care professional–patient relationship. The last three ways arise out of the nature of the modern health care system.

1. Paternalism
Medicine has a long history of paternalism. It was only in the 1960s that issues of autonomy and informed consent were thrust

into the forefront. Old habits, however, die hard. Consequently, many older physicians *and* older patients are more accustomed to a paternalistic style of medical care that emphasizes the physician as the decision maker rather than the patient. Older physicians may think it bizarre medical practice to ask their patients to take responsibility for making treatment choices. Today's elderly patients, long accustomed to paternalistic medical practice, may often be bewildered when told that they must participate in making a treatment choice.

Furthermore, these factors are amplified by the negative conceptions of the elderly which predominate in our society. It is commonly imagined that all elderly persons need looking after, not only physically, but also mentally. This unfortunate misconception promotes paternalistic attitudes towards the elderly as a whole. Even when health care workers are intellectually aware that such misconceptions are mistaken, they can still be motivated by them, even if unconsciously. As an example, physicians, as a matter of course, often consult the younger family members of an elderly patient about the patient's care even when the patient is fully mentally competent. (Notice Dr. Dover's appeal to Mrs. Schaefer's son and daughter.) And elderly patients have often complained to us that the nursing staff treats them, to use the words of one patient, as "senile old biddies who can't think straight or follow even the simplest of directions." This particular patient was also offended by the baby talk and the uninvited first-name familiarity that the nurses used towards her.

These patterns of behavior, which denigrate the personal dignity of elderly persons, will be difficult to alter. The medical profession must confront its paternalistic bias toward the elderly. Efforts must be made by all health care professionals involved in the care of the elderly to gently and non-threateningly guide elderly patients—who are not used to taking an active role in their medical care—in decision making.

2. Difficulty Accepting the Decisions of the Elderly

At some time in a person's life, perhaps in his or her early seventies, a threshold is crossed from middle-age to old-age. This often will be caused by what we may term the "pivotal event." The pivotal event might be a debilitating illness, or the death of a spouse or close friend of the same age group. For whatever reason, the person comes to perceive him- or herself as elderly rather than as middle-aged or even late-middle-aged. The pivotal event provokes the realization that the aging process is progressing towards its culmination. More frequent and more chronic illness is naturally expected, with death as the final event. This transition results in a different perspective on life that someone who has not experienced such a transition may find difficult to understand.

One part of this transition may be that the person comes to see the important events in his or her life as largely in the past rather than the future. (Thomasma 1986) This becomes increasingly true of the "old-old." As there are fewer and fewer future-oriented projects in an elderly person's life, the prolongation of that life becomes less important to him or her than it might once have been. (One must, of course, be careful not to overgeneralize. Some "old-old" persons may indeed have future-oriented projects which they would like to complete before accepting death.) This is not to say that such an elderly person does not value life. It does suggest, however, that such a person might be interested in prolonging life only under acceptable conditions, i.e., with an acceptable quality of life.

Health care professionals must be sensitive to this perspective on life and respect the elderly person's point of view. Sympathetic comprehension of Mrs. Schaefer's stage in life would have made Dr. Dover's duties clearer and more easy to accept.

A distinction must be drawn, however, between a justifiable sadness or acceptance and clinical depression. Clinical depression is a factor that can adversely affect a person's judgment, thereby compromising autonomy. This is a special concern in caring for the elderly since they suffer from a markedly high incidence of depression. But one should not confuse clinical depression with the natural and understandable perspective on life which we have outlined.

3. The Fragmented Nature of Modern Medical Care

Elderly patients are quite likely to suffer from a variety of health-related problems. Consequently, they are often cared for by several different health care professionals. Several physicians, skilled nurses, a dietitian, a physical therapist, and a social worker may all be involved in providing care for an elderly patient.

The large number of different care providers involved produces a fragmentation in health care delivery. This can easily lead to ethically unfortunate consequences. In the same way that a cardiologist may not know what drugs his elderly patient is taking under the direction of a primary care physician or an ophthalmologist, he may not know ethically important information which the primary care physician might know but fails to communicate. This is not unlikely. Since the specialist might see a patient only briefly and episodically, it may be much more convenient (or sometimes even necessary) to proceed by making general assumptions about a patient's value system than to spend seemingly excessive time and energy to gain personal knowledge about a particular patient as a person. Neither is it the case that the primary care physician will necessarily know all the ethically important information. Since the cardiac specialist (or dietitian, nurse, et al.) sees the patient in a different context than a primary care physician, ethically significant information may have been passed from the patient to the specialist of which the primary care physician is unaware.

It is important, therefore, to try to increase the continuity of patient care for the elderly. Specialists should, whenever possible, take the time to talk with patients about value systems and aspirations. They should also consult closely with a patient's primary care physician about such matters. And primary care physicians should be vigorous in sharing and soliciting ethically significant information with specialists as well as nursing staff and other members of the team. And, as noted in chapter 1, it is the responsibility of the primary care physician to ascertain the patient's wishes on a regular basis, for example, as a part of the regular annual examination. This information should be included in arranging referrals or transmitting information to other treating physicians.

4. The Bureaucratic Nature of Institutions

As the modern health care system has grown in complexity, so it has also grown bureaucratically. The health care bureaucracy is designed to work for the advancement of patient care on the whole. It should come as no surprise, however, that the individuality of patients can sometimes mean that the bureaucracy works against their welfare. An example of this can be seen in the case of Mr. Campbell, described in the preceding chapter. Though his primary care physician knew full well that Mr. Campbell opposed

CPR or prolonged ventilation, the structure and regulations of the hospital, designed for patient welfare, dictated that resuscitation be performed. The ICU team intervened to continue Mr. Campbell's life despite the information provided by his primary care physician that Mr. Campbell opposed such measures.

We do not mean to suggest that health care professionals should ignore such rules or that health care institutions should abolish them. Adherence to these rules is usually best for the institution, the health care professional, and the patient. We do mean to suggest, however, that persons designing such policies must keep in mind the ways in which such rules might run counter to a patient's interests and how, if at all possible, to minimize such conflicts.

5. The Fear of Litigation

We live in a very litigious society. This is especially true of the generation which is now often the family involved in the care of elderly patients. Since these middle-aged offspring are far more litigious than their elderly parents, the health care professional may be tempted to honor their wishes even when they run counter to the wishes of the elderly patient. This is especially true when matters of life-saving treatment are involved. The elderly patient may express a wish to avoid some life-saving but invasive and non-curing procedure. The family, on the other hand, may insist that such treatment be rendered and threaten the physician with a lawsuit if he or she does otherwise. Under such circumstances, the physician may well be tempted to acquiesce to the family's wishes in order to avoid legal entanglement, even though it is clear that doing so is contrary to the *patient's* wishes. It is very important, then, that health care professionals keep in mind they are providing care *for the patient*. They have an ethical duty to keep the patient's best interest in mind. (See also Younger and Jackson [1980], and Ruddick [1980].)

Health care professionals have a moral duty to promote the autonomy of their competent patients. This duty should come before inclinations to bow to contrary wishes of the family or the medical staff. Except in the most extreme circumstances (such as when doing so would pose a significant direct threat to innocent third parties), the health care professional has an ethical obligation to accept the settled wishes of the patient. This can, however, be difficult to do. Preconceptions on the part of elderly patients as well as health care professionals can work against the exercise of patient autonomy. And certain aspects of the health care system can also work to the detriment of patients' moral autonomy. Furthermore, the health care professional may find it psychologically difficult to accept a patient's wishes because of the nature of medical education. But the health care professional who is sensitive to these common obstacles to respect for the autonomy of the elderly patient can make a positive difference for the humanity of patients.

Permutations

> 1. Suppose that instead of indicating competency, Dr. Dover's assessment of Mrs. Schaefer suggested she was suffering from depression or schizophrenia.

Health care professionals have a moral obligation to respect the autonomy of their patients. However, if a patient is suffering from depression or some other kind of mental impairment, he or she is not necessarily expressing an autonomous decision. Therefore, though health care professionals may learn information which is important from discussion with such a patient, they are not strictly obliged to acquiesce to choices expressed under such compromised circumstances.

> 2. Suppose that instead of the family members' supporting Mrs. Schaefer's decision they insisted that surgery be performed, even if it required waiting until Mrs. Dover lost consciousness and thus became "incompetent."

The primary ethical obligation of health care professionals is to their patients. As we discuss in chapter 3, there is *some* obligation to the family. Nevertheless, in this instance, where the patient's choice represents no direct harm to or burden upon the family, the obligation to respect the patient's autonomous choice is paramount. Mrs. Schaefer should be allowed her choice.

> 3. Suppose that there is dissension among the members of the health care team. The nurse for the case, for example, may object strongly and threaten to take the matter to the hospital administration.

Even the well functioning health care team will face disagreement from time to time. To minimize alienation and foster teamwork, the team should have a process through which such disagreement is considered. Ethical reservations or objections, when unvoiced or ignored, may lead to more serious health care delivery problems in the future. For two reasons, such disagreement should be acknowledged and dealt with. (a) The dissenter might be right. He or she might see something in the case which the other team members haven't been able to recognize. (b) Dissenting members will work far more enthusiastically and happily with the team if they know that their ethical opinions or beliefs at least have been acknowledged and discussed.

Finally, if a member of the team has a persistent, unresolvable, and serious ethical disagreement with the rest of the team, knowing so may facilitate the move of that team member to a team more in keeping with his or her ethical convictions.

> 4. Suppose that Mrs. Schaefer, instead of living alone, is the sole caretaker for two young grandchildren, the parents having been killed in an automobile accident some years before. Would it still be right to allow her to die?

In similar cases, the state has argued that it has an interest in Mrs. Schaefer's life. This is because Mrs. Schaefer would be considered to have *enforceable* social or moral obligations to other persons. That is, she would have obligations which society has the right to compel her to fulfil, in this case an obligation to support dependent offspring. If the health care professional acquiesced to Mrs. Schaefer's choice, he or she could then be considered morally responsible for direct and significant harm to innocent third parties. In such cases, it is wisest to err on the side of life. If there is sufficient time to consult an institutional ethics committee or hospital lawyer, doing so is highly recommended.

B. The Incompetent Patient

The Case of Mrs. Kovel

Mrs. J. Kovel is a childless widow, 84 years of age, who has not seen a physician for three years following the removal of an adenocarcinoma of the bowel. Her lawyer, who is a family friend and holds power of attorney, sought a "general" medical evaluation, despite Mrs. Kovel's denials, for her declining mental status and as part of a responsible program of follow-up care of her tumor. Dr. Winston's evaluation corroborated the decline in mental status and established criteria consistent with the diagnosis of Alzheimer's disease. The screening tests strongly suggested the possibility of recurrent bowel cancer and a potentially obstructing lesion was subsequently found on barium enema. The patient refused prophylactic surgery. Dr. Winston strongly believed that Mrs. Kovel was not competent to understand the implications of her decision; the lawyer, although he understood the rationale and agreed with Dr. Winston, questioned the wisdom of the operation in an elderly woman; the hospital was uncomfortable in allowing surgery even if she could consent; and the surgical team felt the absolute need for a responsible party to determine resuscitation status and guide decision making should complications arise postoperatively.

Discussion

As we noted at the beginning of this chapter, a significant percentage of the elderly suffer from some mental impairment. Furthermore, there is a direct correlation between increasing age and increasing incidence of mental dysfunction. Since the incompetent patient is, by definition, unable to exercise autonomy (except in the sense of previously stated wishes or documents such as the Living Will), it becomes problematic to think of our primary ethical duty as that of promoting the autonomy of these patients. Instead, our duty of beneficence comes to the foreground and it becomes not only acceptable, but *proper,* to act paternalistically toward the patient for the sake of his or her own welfare (though not toward the family). The loss of competency drastically alters the ethical complexion of the provider-patient relationship. A different system of moral obligations must come into play.

Before proceeding to our discussion of the ethical significance of incompetency, however, there are important, and all too often overlooked, distinctions between different kinds of incompetency. The medical profession does distinguish between organic and inorganic, reversible and irreversible dementia. But what we are concerned with here, as it has important ethical implications, is a distinction between different kinds of skills.

One sense in which a person can be incompetent is with respect to property. The person in question may not pay his or her electric or telephone bills. He or she may be unable to keep food available. He or she may give money away in a manner that seems irresponsible. A judicial proceeding can be initiated by family members or by the state to determine if the person in question is disposing of his or her property in a manner which indicates a lack of "sound mind." Medical staff may, on occasion, be called upon to offer their assessment in such proceedings. For further discussion of these matters, see Schmidt (1985) and Kapp and Bigot (1985, chapter 8).

Another sense of incompetence, and one which is of central concern here, is the person's inability to make and act upon rational decisions. This may be termed incompetence with respect to the person. When this kind of incompetency is present, then the kind of moral-rational autonomy which ethics is keen to protect in individuals is absent. If a person cannot in principle understand what is at issue, it is meaningless to expect him or her to make reasoned choices.

There is a regrettable tendency of many in the health care professions to assume that if an elderly person is incompetent in the sense of not being able to manage the daily business of life, then he or she is also incompetent to make decisions concerning medical treatment options. The failure to distinguish these two different kinds of incompetency means that patients who are incompetent with regard to property only, but who still possess a clear conception of the self as well as an ability to make sensible choices concerning treatment, are frequently deprived of their moral right to make important decisions concerning their own fates.

Paternalistic medical decision-making procedures are clearly appropriate in dealing with those who are incompetent with respect to person. The same is not the case, though, for those who are only incompetent with respect to property. The remainder of this discussion directs itself, therefore, to the issues raised by incompetence with respect to person.

B.1 The Ethical Significance of the Loss of Competency

Since there is an absence of rational will on the part of incompetent persons, it becomes appropriate to treat them in a paternalistic manner. That is, on the basis of the duties of beneficence and non-maleficence, we must take responsibility for decision making in the same fashion that parents make important decisions on behalf of their children. Paternalism is immoral when it violates a person's autonomy, but since in the case of the irreversibly demented elderly there is no autonomy, there can be no such violation.

There can be, however, a great deal of controversy over what this acceptance of paternalistic responsibility commits us to. James Rachels (1986) and Tristram Engelhardt (1986) have argued that when rationality becomes absent, the patient is no longer a "person." Hence we no longer have the same sorts of moral obligations toward them that we do have toward *persons*. It becomes morally legitimate to withhold treatment from a profoundly demented patient which might be morally required for a mentally sound patient, simply because of the dementia.

Such theories may be difficult to accept because they run counter to deeply held feelings. It *might* be true that in the case of the persistently vegetative, irreversibly comatose or higher-brain-dead patients we can come to understand them over time as no longer fully "persons." But such beliefs are very difficult to accept with respect to the demented. This is, we believe, because most people have deeply felt moral sentiments, through a kind of sympathy, with such individuals. And these sentiments preclude the hasty deletion of such individuals from the list of persons. The individual who lies on the bed in the nursing home, even if hopelessly demented, is still "Mother" or "Father." The social history, bound up with such individuals, particularly in a family context, rightly prevents them from being considered no longer persons. This is not to say, however, that such dementia does not or should never alter what medical decisions are morally appropriate. In the minds of many persons, to prolong the life of such severely demented persons can be more cruel than allowing them to die.

At the other end of the spectrum, Paul Ramsey argues (1970) that since such demented patients are "voiceless," we should never withhold or withdraw any sort of treatment which might keep them alive. Such patients cannot exert their own autonomy, so it is impossible for them to defend themselves. Such things as dialysis, CPR, nutrition, antibiotics, or ICU care should never be withheld or withdrawn from a patient who is demented. To do so *might* be contrary to what the patient would want if he or she was able to competently express such a wish.

Both of these views strike us as extreme. The first view does not do justice to the strong moral sentiments which we may feel toward the elderly demented. The second view ignores the fact that there are many circumstances in which reasonable persons would prefer non-treatment to treatment. Ramsey's position robs the demented elderly of their rights just as effectively as the positions advocated by Rachels and Engelhardt.

We suggest a more moderate way of understanding our ethical obligations toward the irreversibly demented. As autonomy disappears, our duties of beneficence and non-maleficence come more to the forefront. Since we cannot consult with our patients concerning their own conception of their best interests, we must turn to different sources of authority. There are two different sorts of authority.

Advance Directives: The first, and most desirable, is determination of what that particular individual would want if he or she were capable of expressing such a wish. This determination rests upon having information concerning the patient's value systems prior to the loss of competency. Common sources for such information are a Living Will, durable power of attorney, or other such advance directives, or information from someone who was close to the individual, such as close family members, clergy, close friends or neighbors. Since this information concerns the particular value systems of the person in question, it should be considered as an extension of personal autonomy. If the health care provider can ascertain with reasonable certainty what the particular patient would value, it becomes a moral obligation to act upon that knowledge.

Since the expressions of elderly persons when competent are undoubtedly the most reliable report of their particular value systems, it should be clear why we stressed in the previous chapter the physician's responsibility to gather information from patients as a routine aspect of patient care. The solicitation of such information should not be casually postponed until a crisis comes or until the patient has already lost his or her cognitive capacities. To postpone the gathering of such ethically important patient information is often to place it forever beyond our grasp.

Proxy: The second sort of authority plays a role when there is no reliable way to ascertain what the particular patient in question would have wanted. Under these circumstances the health care provider must rely upon substituted judgment. Legal designation of the appropriate person to take on this role varies from state to state, but the immediate family is often given special consideration.

The ethical ideal, under these conditions, is to determine what a reasonable person would want. One may approach the issue at hand by using sympathetic imagination. Imaginatively placing oneself in the patient's position, one then asks what would I or any such reasonable person prefer to be done?

Mrs. Kovel, we may recall, opposed surgery to remove the obstructive lesion in her bowel. Conversations with Mrs. Kovel raised doubts in the physician's mind concerning her competency. If Mrs. Kovel was incompetent with respect to her person, then it became the physician's moral duty to promote her best interests on her behalf, rather than necessarily accepting her own stated opinions.

The physician's first task, then, was to identify what course of action would be in Mrs. Kovel's best interests, as understood by a reasonable, mentally competent person. What the physician sensibly did was to identify the different possible courses of action and their probable outcomes.

(1) Not operating at all almost inevitably led to one outcome—a painful and unpleasant death by intestinal obstruction.

(2) Operating upon Mrs. Kovel had two distinct possibilities. (a) First, her advanced age increased the statistical probability of undesirable complications from surgery. Though not highly likely, it was still a significant possibility that she might die from the surgery. (b) Second, it was quite likely that, if the surgery went well and since she did not suffer from any other threatening physical illnesses, she would live several more years before dying from some unrelated and perhaps less painful disease.

Since a painful death was almost inevitable in the near future if the surgery was not done, it seemed to the physician unreasonable to avoid the surgery on account of the risks to Mrs. Kovel. What did she really have to lose? On the other hand, the surgery did offer a reasonably good chance of several more years of a comfortable, if demented, life. Consequently, the physician believed that a reasonable person would opt for the surgery.

B.2 Identifying the Decision Maker

It is important to recognize here that not all reasonable persons will always come up with the same decisions, even when provided with the same information. Since there may be differences of opinion among family members and health care providers about what to do, it is imperative that the health care system (be it the hospital, nursing home, or private physician's office) have a policy designating who assumes decision making responsibility in cases where there are no clear and relevant advance directives.

As noted above, different states have slightly different policies on these matters, but for the most part preference is given to the closest competent family member in identifying a decision maker for an incompetent person. The physician is expected to play an important consulting role, however. In cases where the physician, as the leader of the health care team, strongly disagrees with the designated guardian, arbitration should be sought at a higher level—perhaps first an internal committee, and then (failing all else), the judiciary.

We have argued that when the elderly patient cannot exercise true autonomy we should paternalistically act to protect the patient's interests. This is done by determining what a reasonable person would want under the relevant circumstances. As even the most casual reader of medical ethics will know, medical ethics literature is in virtually unanimous opinion on the matter. However, as the medical practitioner will know, it can be very difficult to determine what this hypothetical "reasonable" person would want. Physicians may disagree with other medical staff; the health care team may disagree with the family; and the family may well be in conflict itself.

Not only may our particular relations with a patient affect what we see as "reasonable," but our age may itself be a factor.

Will a 27-year-old resident physician in internal medicine have the same world view as a "reasonable" 84-year-old nursing home patient? Will the 59-year-old physician, worried about aging and retirement, have the same acceptance of old age as a bed-bound 93-year-old who has lost a spouse and whose offspring live far away? Or will an exuberantly athletic 30-year-old physician have the same notion of a "minimal acceptable quality of life" as an 80-year-old arthritic candidate for hip surgery?

We believe that it is quite natural that our approach toward living will evolve through different age brackets and life events. We suggest that the ethically best understanding of what a "reasonable" person would want should be taken to mean what a competent person *of the same age bracket and life outlook* would want. Young health care professionals may greatly overestimate their ability to know what their elderly patients would want.

It would make sense, therefore, for health care professionals caring for incompetent elderly patients to actively consult with competent elderly patients. For lacking prior directive from the incompetent patient or clear knowledge on the part of the family, other competent elderly patients are probably the best guide to "what the patient would want if competent." This might be done by having a consulting committee in a nursing home or retirement community, composed of select competent residents. In the hospital setting, elderly community members might be asked to serve on such committees. And in ambulatory practice, the physician may want to develop a "community of elders" for the purpose of consultation.

The irreversible absence of a person's rational will alters the ethical complexion of the patient-provider relationship. If there is evidence of the patient's true wishes, such as can be found in advance directives, then such evidence should be considered as an extension of the patient's autonomy and should be respected. In the absence of such information, since there is no longer any meaningful autonomy to preserve or promote, it becomes the health care professional's ethical obligation to act in coordination with others to make decisions on the patient's behalf. This is morally proper medical paternalism. The difficulty, as we have seen, is in ascertaining what a "reasonable" person would want done—or not done. Our closing suggestion is that the elderly themselves are the most valuable, and most underused, resource in determining such issues.

Permutations

1. In cases involving dangerous treatment, judicial review for incompetent patients is frequently mandated. It sometimes happens that even in cases where the appointed guardian and physician agree on the ethically proper choice, a judge (for whatever reason) might overrule them, dictating his own choice. What should one do then?

Judges are not perfectly wise. If the stakes are high enough, the appointed guardian and the physician may refile the case with another judge.

2. Suppose Mrs. Kovel was "tragically demented." That is, her life is very unpleasant for her because of her physical and mental debility. Should this count as a reason for withholding treatment?

We believe that the patient's quality of life does play a role in the ethically proper determination of treatment decisions. One element of quality of life assessments is mental status and whether it adversely affects the patient's well-being. This is not to suggest that mental ability itself is a criterion for non-treatment. To use it as such would be unethically discriminatory. For more on this matter, see chapter 6.

C. The Marginally Competent Patient

The Case of Dr. Reed and Mrs. Malone

Mrs. Malone, 70, seems quite normal in casual conversation. She also performs adequately on mental screening tests. And she can tell Dr. Reed what she needs to do. Nevertheless, Mrs. Malone does not act in her own best interest.

Mrs. Malone has sprue. Whenever she eats wheat

products she suffers from severe diarrhea which leads to hypocalcemia and malnutrition. So why does she insist on eating Wonderbread on occasions, maintaining it is good for her? Why hasn't she learned from her eight hospitalizations within the past year?

Mrs. Malone's physicians, headed by Dr. Reed, have prescribed magnesium and calcium supplements. Mrs. Malone can tell Dr. Reed the appropriate dosage and schedules; she can repeat why she needs the supplements; and she tells you that she wants to take them. So why does she always have an excuse for either not buying the medications or for not taking them? Unless brought to the office by the social worker, Mrs. Malone does not keep her scheduled office visits.

Her income from a pension and Social Security is adequate to meet her needs. Yet she does not consistently pay her rent or utility bills. She has the eviction notices and letters threatening discontinuation of service in neat piles along with her own correspondence. Her checkbook is accurately balanced and reveals that she donates a substantial portion of her monies to environmental charities and television evangelists.

During her most recent hospitalization, the health care team caring for Mrs. Malone sought a psychiatric evaluation, wondering if institutionalization might be for Mrs. Malone's benefit. The evaluation concluded that Mrs. Malone was probably in an early phase of Alzheimer's disease and that her major deficiencies were in judgment, reasoning, and personal hygiene, and that she had a mild memory impairment. But it was not thought that these deficiencies were severe enough to warrant the label "incompetent."

Concerned that Mrs. Malone's health and well-being were increasingly endangered, Dr. Reed led the health care team in an effort to obtain guardianship. The judge, however, after hearing testimony from Mrs. Malone, ruled that she was competent. Guardianship was denied and Mrs. Malone was discharged after several further days of hospitalization.

Discussion

In cases where a patient is clearly competent or incompetent it is relatively easy to delineate our ethical duties. In caring for a fully competent patient, respect for the patient's autonomy is a very strong duty. In caring for an incompetent patient, respect for autonomy has little or no relevance and the duties of beneficence and non-maleficence become most important. But health care professionals who care for the elderly will be aware that many of their patients suffer from *degrees* of dementia. Impairment from Alzheimer's disease or multi-infarct dementia, varieties of dementia to which the elderly are disproportionately susceptible, may be nearly imperceptible at first, becoming increasingly obvious and severe over a number of years.

This means that the loss of cognitive capacities can happen gradually over a period of years. Hence, for a substantial period of time, the elderly patient suffering from a progressive loss of cognitive function will be neither fully competent nor fully incompetent. Instead, there is a large grey zone in which there are various degrees of *marginal competency.*

Since elderly patients who fall into this grey zone are neither truly competent nor incompetent, the ethical analyses of the health care professional's relationship to competent and incompetent patients offered above are not directly applicable. Though rarely acknowledged, the ethical quandaries raised by the grey zone of marginal competency deserve special ethical discussion. (See Culver CM 1985.)

Suppose, for example, a marginally competent patient refuses a treatment which her physician thinks is to her benefit. Is the physician to be guided by respect for autonomy or by duties of beneficence and non-maleficence? Would violating what autonomy the patient does have be justified on the grounds of beneficence?

How to balance respect for autonomy with duties of beneficence and non-maleficence usually becomes a practical ethical concern under two circumstances: (1) When the patient disagrees with the physician or a family member concerning a procedure, or (2) when the health care team is proposing something where there is more than one medically acceptable course of action and decision-making authority is being sought.

We suggest a kind of balancing act as the most ethically desirable method of deciding how to regard the wishes of the marginally competent patient. If respecting the patient's autonomy does not run a serious risk to the patient's health and well-being, such autonomy as there is ought to be respected. However, if adhering to the patient's voiced wishes would entail a *serious, unreasonable,* and *unnecessary risk,* either through foregone highly beneficial intervention or through intervention of unnecessary risk and little compensating benefit, then the duties of beneficence and non-maleficence ought to be seen as of greater importance. The idea behind this scheme is to extend the benefit of doubt to the marginally competent patient except in those circumstances where the unreasonableness of the patient's voiced wishes are themselves strong evidence of lack of competency. This may be schematically represented as in Figure 1.

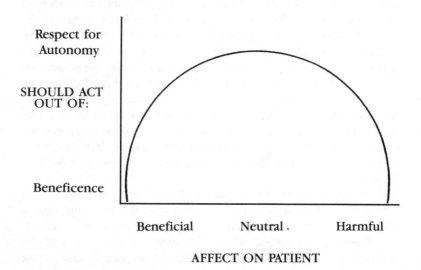

FIGURE 1

The scheme would work in the following way. (1) If a proposed procedure is clearly in the patient's welfare (from the point of view of a reasonable person), but the patient refuses the procedure without offering any sensible explanation, the physician and family should be inclined to override the patient's wishes, seeking protective guardianship if necessary. (2) If the outcome of the proposed procedure is not clear-cut, but is probably beneficial, the physician and family should heed the patient's wishes, even if they disagree. (3) If the patient wishes a procedure performed which is of no benefit, but is rather of potentially serious harm, the physician and family should override the patient's wishes. While decisions in (1) and (3) may infringe upon a patient's autonomy, the action is justified by an overriding concern for the patient's welfare coupled with serious doubts concerning the patient's competency. Circumstance (2), however, tolerates the risk of some harm or lost benefit as an acceptable risk in the effort to respect the patient's rights.

One thing that must be kept in mind is that if the medical team is considering overriding the wishes of a marginally competent elderly patient, they must consider in their deliberations not only the effect upon the patient of the specific medical procedure or activity in question, but also the effect of overriding the patient's wishes, i.e., of negating the patient's autonomy. The marginally competent patient is in the unfortunate position of being a legitimate candidate for being overridden while at the same time being sufficiently cognitively functional to recognize the invalidation of his or her autonomy. This can be particularly distressing to the elderly person, who is quite likely already sensitive to subtle mental changes (such as loss of memory). The depression and alienation which such an intervention might cause, therefore, must be factored against the positive consequences of the proposed intervention.

In general terms, the greater and more certain the potential overall benefit or harm, the more we should feel compelled to override the adverse wishes of the marginally competent patient.

The case of Dr. Reed and Mrs. Malone illustrates many of the difficult questions raised in caring for the marginally competent patient. To begin with, notice that the medical staff is ambivalent concerning Mrs. Malone's mental status. Mrs. Malone "performs adequately" on the mental status screening tests. And the psychiatric evaluation concluded that, though she was in an early phase of Alzheimer's disease, her deficiencies were not severe enough "to warrant the label 'incompetent.' " Despite these evaluations, the health care team, led by Dr. Reed, decided to seek guardianship through the courts, since they felt that Mrs. Malone could not be trusted to look after her own welfare. This ambivalence on the part of the health care professionals involved is a result of Mrs. Malone's marginal mental status.

Dr. Reed's approach to the problem reflects what we have outlined as circumstance (3). That is, the patient insists upon some procedure or engaging in some practice which is of no benefit and which is quite probably of potentially severe harm. Dr. Reed's judgment in this instance was that, without supervision, Mrs. Malone was more than likely going to cause considerable harm to herself. Furthermore, it is not a harm which the patient could be said to have elected to suffer, since she could not understand that there was a connection between eating white bread and ending up in the hospital. Dr. Reed concluded that the threat was clear enough and serious enough to warrant overriding the limited competence which Mrs. Malone possessed. In this specific case, there were no family members or close associates to whom Dr. Reed could turn for further information, nor a caretaker who could help ensure Mrs. Malone's adherence to patterns of behavior appropriate to her medical circumstances. Consequently, Dr. Reed led the team in seeking judicial guardianship.

We suggest that Dr. Reed acted in an ethically acceptable manner, though she might have been more sure of herself if she had approached the case using a conscious decision procedure involving the kinds of considerations which we have outlined. Furthermore, as mentioned, there is the possibility of bringing the case before a different judge, where a different decision might be reached.

As events actually developed, the judge presiding over the case refused to deem Mrs. Malone incompetent. The law, by its nature, is geared for either/or categories. Thus it is not too surprising that the judge classified Mrs. Malone as competent. On another occasion, before a different judge, the decision might well go the other direction.

The medical team, we believe, is guessing when her next admission will be.

Permutations

   1. Suppose that the family of a marginally competent patient feels strongly one way or the other about therapy choices. Should their feelings play a role in decision making?

The opinions of the family should be taken into account in the following ways. (a) If the proposed treatment would impose a great burden upon the family (such as chronic home care) then that should be considered. (b) As in the case of incompetent patients, the family can be a valuable source of information about the patient. They may have knowledge concerning the patient's value systems that is unavailable to the physician. Such information might help the health care professional better discern the gradations of competency as well as the more settled value systems of the patient. This information can clearly play a significant role in balancing between compromised autonomy and the patient's well-being.

D. Non-adherence versus Non-compliance

The Case of Dr. Barker and Mrs. Krieger

"Mrs. Krieger had a bad combination of problems: She did not want to take medications, but she suffered from hypertension. As a result, she finally developed severe congestive heart failure.

"Our team was first asked to see Mrs. Krieger in her apartment by her son, Michael, whose faith in his mother's physician was steadily waning. She had been admitted to the hospital three times within the last two months and six times already that year. Michael showed us the medications she was supposed to take and assured us that they were administered when he visited twice each day.

"We found it difficult to believe that her hypertension could have gotten so out of control if she had been taking the prescribed medications. Our suspicions were confirmed when the medical student with me found pills among the sheets, under the bed, and in the wastebasket nearby.

"When confronted with this, Mrs. Krieger was not at all apologetic. She said she "didn't believe in all that medicine," and felt that it was the concrete and linoleum floor that sapped her strength.

"We began by asking her about her prejudices against medications and found that she was most distressed by the large number of tablets required by her regimen. Some of her complaints were clearly the result of her diuretics which, because of her immobility, caused her to be incontinent. A few other complaints could be traced to side effects common to her drugs.

"We began to search for changes we might make to lessen these disagreeable effects. The massive edema precluded the withdrawal of her diuretics, but a bedside commode compensated for her immobility. In order to adjust to her aversion to numerous tablets, we had the pharmacy combine as many drugs as possible and used elixirs when available.

"She seemed amenable to this restructuring, and we left quite pleased with ourselves."

Discussion

For a variety of reasons, a significant percentage of elderly persons do not carry out the treatment instructions of their physicians. It is precisely that there are a variety of reasons that this matter needs discussion. A distinction needs to be recognized between two quite different reasons why elderly patients may fail to follow a prescribed regimen.

Non-adherence

Mrs. Krieger represents a patient who has willfully *chosen* not to adhere with a prescribed regimen. It is not because of a lack of understanding or forgetfulness that she does not adhere to her treatment. Rather, it is because she finds the regimen objectionable.

We may easily understand why this is a problem in caring for the elderly in particular. As they become elderly, they suffer from more and more medical conditions at the same time. These conditions, often of a chronic nature, are frequently treated by drugs or other such therapy. The elderly may face the prospect of taking a large number of drugs at the same time for an indefinite stretch of time. Or they may be required to engage in physical therapy which they find painful and intrusive in their settled style of life.

Given these circumstances, the elderly patient may decide that the regimen is just not worth the trouble. This has become known as "patient non-adherence." The patient *chooses* not to comply with the prescribed therapy.

If the health care professional is able to discover this behavior and recognize the motivation of the elderly patient, it becomes possible to deal with the situation constructively. In this case, Dr. Barker managed to discover the non-adherence as well as the reasons for the behavior. Hence, he was able to reformulate Mrs. Krieger's regimen into a form that she found significantly less objectionable. If he had simply assumed that it was because she couldn't understand the regimen (an assumption grounded on our society's negative conceptions of the elderly), then all the education that he might give her would not have made any difference. To make a difference, it is necessary to recognize and respect the reasons for non-adherence, negotiating a mutually acceptable compromise.

With the non-adherent patient, therefore, the most constructive approach involves (a) educating the patient on the importance of adherence, (b) compromising with the patient to reach a regimen that will be acceptable, and (c) enjoining the patient to adhere to the agreed-upon regimen.

Non-compliance

A different reason for failure to follow a prescribed regimen, however, is lack of understanding or lack of memory. This reason is called "non-compliance." Here the patient *wants* to follow the prescribed treatment, but because of mental (or, in some cases, physical) reasons is unable.

The health care professional must realize that in these cases admonishing the patient to follow the regimen is not helpful and, perhaps, might even prove counter-productive. The solution in these sorts of cases is (a) educating the patient better and (b) simplifying the treatment if at all possible. This may result in giving up some of the therapy which the health care professional might think valuable. But keep in mind that if the result of absolutely full therapy is non-compliance, then reduced therapy may well be more beneficial to the patient. Some compromise between desired therapy and the abilities of the patient may be required.

Annotated Bibliography

Kapp MB, and Bigot A. *Geriatrics and the Law,* New York: Springer Publishing, 1985.
This text provides a solid overview of the legal issues in-

volved in caring for the elderly, including competency and consent, limited treatment, and euthanasia.

References

Cassell E. "The nature of suffering and the goals of medicine," *New England Journal of Medicine* 306:639–45 (1982).

Christie RJ, and Hoffmaster B. *Ethical Issues in Family Medicine,* New York: Oxford University Press, 1986.

Culver CM. "The Clinical Determination of Competence," in *Legal and Ethical Aspects of Health Care for the Elderly* (ed. by Kapp MB, Pies HE, and Doudera AE), Ann Arbor: Health Administration Press, 1985.

Engelhardt HT. *The Foundations of Bioethics,* New York: Oxford University Press, 1986.

Kapp MB, and Bigot A. *Geriatrics and the Law,* New York: Springer Publishing, 1985.

Katzman R, Terry RD, Bedell SE. "Senile Dementia and Related Disorders," from *Alzheimer's Disease,* New York: Raven Press, 1978, pp. 323–26.

Rachels J. *The End of Life,* Oxford: Oxford University Press, 1986.

Ramsey P. *The Patient as Person,* New Haven: Yale University Press, 1970.

Ruddick W. "Commentary on Family Wishes and Patient Autonomy," *Hastings Center Report,* 1980, p. 22.

Schmidt WC. "Guardianship: Public and Private," in *Legal and Ethical Aspects of Health Care for the Elderly* (ed. by Kapp MB, Pies HE, and Doudera AE), Ann Arbor: Health Administration Press, 1985.

Younger SJ, and Jackson DL. "Commentary on Family Wishes and Patient Autonomy," *Hastings Center Report,* 1980, pp. 21–22.

CHAPTER 3

The Family

The Case of Mrs. Castle

The surgeon finally appeared at the doorway, hesitated, and then stepped into the waiting room with the bad news: mother's biopsies were positive. The tumor had obviously spread.

Mr. Castle looked resignedly at his wife, who obviously shared the sense of grief for Mrs. Castle as a mother-in-law and as another woman. Their daughter, Lisa, began to cry, and her parents moved away from the surgeon to comfort her.

Later, the family met with Mrs. Castle, who stated, "I want to go home. I want to die in my own bed, like my mother did. Laura, you *will* take care of me, won't you?"

The elder Mrs. Castle instinctively knew that this was her last illness and prayed that her end would come swiftly. She also knew that she was in competition for attention with her spiteful granddaughter, of whom she was already quite resentful. The girl was not having an easy time of adolescence, sampling drugs, acting rebelliously, and doing poorly in school. She was now remarkably subdued, restrained like an angry cat, sitting coiled in the corner of the hospital room.

The couple turned to the surgeon who, despite his initial demeanor, seemed very hopeful that chemotherapy and radiation would give her another couple of good years, "maybe three to five." He was like a judge passing sentence, glad that a difficult trial was approaching an end. They, however, saw only a prolonged course of recurrence, progressive disability, and eventually death. A tough road to travel in any case, but with problems with Lisa, it seemed overwhelming.

"We think," ventured Mr. Castle, "that mother would be better off in a nursing home. We'll visit often. . . but we just can't handle her at home."

Discussion

The scene is not uncommon, but from the point of view of contemporary medical ethics it raises some serious questions. The patient, a 75-year-old woman, is quite competent, yet her family, in a non-emergency situation, has been informed of her medical condition before she is even aware of it. Has her right to physician-patient confidentiality been violated? Has the family shirked an obligation which they have? Would the physician be betraying the elder Mrs. Castle if he, against his hopes, agreed to place her in a nursing home?

The bulk of contemporary medical ethics focuses either on the health care provider's relationship to the patient or society's relationship to the patient. Little attention is paid to the everyday clinical practice of involving the family of the patient in both deciding among treatment options and providing health care. Hence, it is often the case that health care professionals find themselves in an ethical triad involving the patient and family. This is particularly true in the case of elderly patients where, because of the nature of chronic care, families often ask or are asked to play a significant role.

We must, therefore, examine how relationships within the family affect the ethical complexion of the patient-provider relationship.

Family Bonds
In order to understand why it is ethically proper frequently to engage the family in the care of an elderly patient, let us draw a schematic picture of a "healthy" or "well-functioning" family. Four points should be made.

1) *There is a mutuality of interests.* The well-functioning family can be understood as a mixture of individualism and unity.

Each member of the family is recognized and encouraged to think and act as an individual—that is, a healthy family encourages individual autonomy. On the other hand, it is distorting to view family members as entirely discrete individuals. Family members naturally develop familial bonds with each other. By a process of sympathetic interest ("fellow feeling") each family member takes a real interest in the welfare of the others. The happiness of one member also becomes the happiness of others. And any misfortune which befalls one also touches upon the others.

This mutuality of interest means that each member of a healthy family wants good for the other family members, since by extension that would also be good for the self; and each wants to avoid or prevent ill from befalling the others, since by extension ill to them would be an ill to the self. When a family member, such as an elderly parent, becomes ill, the family as a whole wants that elderly person to become better (or at least to be kept as well as possible).

2) *There is deep personal knowledge.* In a healthy family, the various members, by having lived together and by sharing interests, will have developed extensive personal knowledge about each other. They will know each other's likes and dislikes, hopes and fears, ambitions and aspirations. The family, therefore, can act as a valuable resource for the health care professional in evaluating the elderly patient and in planning treatment and therapy.

3) *The family can play a positive role in health care.* The family can play a significant role in several ways.

- First, they can reinforce healthy behavior patterns. An involved and supportive family can ensure that balanced meals are eaten regularly; that physical exercise is performed; and that mental stimulation is provided.
- Second, they can facilitate recuperation. By ensuring that the patient adheres to the prescribed therapy, including physical activity, the family can assist in the healing process. Or if the disease or incapacity is chronic, they can help maintain as much independence and health as is feasible.
- Third, by providing emotional support, the family can foster an attitude in the elderly individual that encourages healing and health.

4) *There is always a potential for patient-family conflict of interest.* Even in the healthy family where there is a deep mutual-

ity of interests, there may arise a conflict of interest between the elderly individual and the rest of the family. In some instances, the individual in question may be willing to sacrifice personal benefit for the good of the whole. But this issue can only be raised if we are willing to acknowledge the potential for such conflict. And, as should be obvious to the health care professional, many families deviate substantially from such an idealized model, such that mutuality of interest is at best very weak.

Since health care professionals promote the interests of the patient as their moral duty, they share certain goals with the family as a whole. How they work towards these goals, though, will be quite different. The health care professional will make use of specialized training in medicine, nursing, social work, and so on. The family, on the other hand, is far better at providing such things as emotional support and a nurturing home environment. Since the health care professional and the family share goals *and* achieve those goals through different but complementary ways, there *should* be cooperation between them. Nevertheless, as we have noted, conflicts of interest can arise between patient and family.

Let us consider, now, how these potential conflicts between the individual and the family can raise ethical complexities for the practicing health care professional.

Confidentiality

There are many reasons why the health care professional may want to share patient information with family members. But, we must ask, what would count as ethically justifiable reasons for divulging patient information? In the case of Mrs. Castle, was her confidentiality with the surgeon unethically violated?

In the case of the incompetent patient, the health care professional will need to identify some person (or group of persons) who may authoritatively speak for the incapacitated patient. For reasons discussed above, ethics recommends that (except under unusual circumstances) the patient's family ought to be allowed this role. Also, family members may necessarily be involved in day-to-day activities of patient care. If so, it is only fair that they understand not only what they need to do, but why.

The matter becomes somewhat more complicated in the case of mentally competent patients. The family, even if not directly involved in patient care, may have a sincere interest in the patient's condition and progress. This interest is not one of idle curiosity, but rather motivated by deeply felt affection for the patient (who is likely a parent or spouse). Furthermore, if the family is kept abreast of the patient's status, it is possible that they can help the patient. Families can often ensure that an elderly relative with impaired mobility has adequate food supplies in the dwelling. They can help ensure that necessary errands are performed. And, perhaps most importantly, they can emotionally support the patient in a way that maximizes the patient's overall well-being.

The sincere love and care which many family members will have for their elderly will itself encourage the health care professional to share information. This is especially true as a patient may approach death and the physician may feel the obligation to prepare family members for the event and its aftermath.

The ethical complexities of this triad (provider-patient-family) pose a serious challenge to popular notions of physician-patient confidentiality. While most medical ethicists argue that the health care provider's ethical obligation is strictly to the patient, and recommend a strict version of physician-patient confidentiality, some ethicists argue that a deeper understanding of the family as a unit dictates a modified notion of confidentiality. This point has been most forcefully argued by Christie and Hoffmaster in their *Ethical Issues in Family Medicine* (1986).

As we argued in chapter 1, we think that the wisest course of action is for the health care professional, particularly the physician, to clarify with the patient the scope of confidentiality with respect to family members. This should be done at the outset of treatment, at each subsequent annual exam, and again at any significant turn of events.

This should not be taken lightly as a quick question and answer session. The patient who readily agrees that all information concerning his or her health may be shared with family members should be reminded of the various kinds of information that might become involved. Analogously, when a patient requests that all information be kept confidential, the health care professional ought to explore the reasons for this request, particularly if one does not suspect antipathy between the patient and family.

Given the variety of ways in which a supportive family can promote the independence, comfort, and overall well-being of an elderly patient, we think it ethically appropriate for the physician to encourage such a patient to agree to the sharing of a great deal of patient information with close family members. This does not mean that all information should or need be divulged. The physician and patient may agree that highly personal information, such as sexual matters, be kept strictly confidential.

Finally, as noted in chapter 1, health care professionals should not assume that they know the preferences of their patients in these matters without explicitly discussing them.

The Scope of the Family's Authority

Although there is not unanimity of opinion, a number of recent legal decisions have vested decision-making authority in the immediate family when a patient is mentally incompetent. Our discussion in this chapter has, we hope, shown that there are good moral grounds for such a practice. Just as there are legal limits to the authority which a family member may exert over one of its elderly members, so there are also *moral* limits. In the case of competent individuals, both law and morality recognize the general precedence of patient autonomy over family wishes. In the case of incompetent persons, both law and morality place a great deal of authority (though not absolute authority) in the family. And, though the law prefers to see things in black or white, mental competency in the elderly is often a question of gradations of grey. Therefore, there must be some moral process of weighing the value of the marginally competent patient's autonomy.

As a way of understanding the moral scope of family authority over patient care decisions, we suggest the following model. Assuming a healthy family relationship (i.e., the family is not malicious towards the elderly person, does not abuse him or her, but does have a loving interest in the patient's welfare), the family's moral authority is negligible when the patient is competent, and gradually increases as the patient progresses through marginal competency to incompetency. The family has greatest moral authority when the patient is mentally incompetent, but this authority is still not absolute (in order that the state may protect against gross abuse of the individual by the family).

The ethical rationale behind this model is that as the patient loses competency, he or she loses authority to that degree. Yet, in order to prevent the abuse of vulnerable individuals, the state does not give absolute authority to the family, even when the patient is hopelessly demented or comatose. If the health care professional believes that the family is acting contrary to the interests of the elderly person, appeal may be made to the judiciary to override the decisions or actions of the family.

Limits to Family Authority

In the discussion so far, we have assumed a "healthy" family, which is only an idealized model. As the health care professional will be all too well aware, however, many elderly persons do not have this type of relationship with their family. Instead of acting out of loving care and devotion for the elderly family member, many families may act out of selfish motives. They may keep an elderly family member at home, contrary to the health care professional's recommendation, in order to have access to the elderly person's income, such as a social security check. They may want to place the elderly person in a nursing home, not for medical reasons, but because they do not want to bother with him or her. The family may want to keep the elderly member out of institutional care because they do not want to see their potential inheritance spent on expensive extended care. Or they may insist on palliative treatment only, not out of a desire to prevent unnecessary harm to the elderly person, but to hasten his or her death so that the inheritance might be gained that much earlier.

In instances such as these, the family lacks the genuine commitment to the elderly person that the "healthy" family has. Such a family cannot be trusted to have the elderly person's best interests at heart. In such cases, the ethical reasons why we normally invest the family with decision-making authority for the incompetent (or to a degree for the marginally competent) elderly patient are voided.

The health care team must work closely together in such cases if they are to protect the best interests of the elderly person. As health care professionals, their obligation to the elderly patient requires that they identify and document the problem. For by doing so, judicial intervention, wherein a legal guardian may be appointed in place of the family, becomes a plausible option. Without such active intervention by the health care team, it is likely that the elderly who are abused by such families because of their dependent relationship will continue to be abused.

Limits to the Family's Obligations

Traditional models of the provider-patient relationship emphasize the provider's obligation to the patient as an *individual*. That is, the provider is supposed to have an ethical obligation to have the *patient's* best interest in mind when designing and providing care. This view, however, must be regarded as greatly oversimplified since it ignores the fact that health care, especially chronic care of the elderly, can place burdens upon other individuals. Is the health care team shirking its moral duty if it acquiesces to the family's wish to place Mrs. Castle in a nursing home, knowing that Mrs. Castle wants to go home and believing that she would be better off at home? Aren't we frequently told that there is a principle of medical ethics which states, "Above all, do no harm" *(Primum non nocere)?*

The health care professional must be sensitive to the burdens that proposed patient care may place on third parties, particularly the family. In this case, for example, we suggest the health care team would not be guilty of any moral wrongdoing by taking into account the adverse effect of their proposed treatment plan upon the family, even though Mrs. Castle will suffer.

The reason has to do with considerations of *moral justice.* For example, it is unjust to provide an ICU bed to someone who doesn't really need intensive care. Doing so may prevent someone else who genuinely needs intensive care from having access to the unit. It would be an unjust squandering of scarce and valuable resources. As another example, the physician's obligation to confidentiality is overridden by third party interests in the case of highly dangerous and communicable diseases. Hence syphilis and gonorrhea are legally reportable diagnoses. By stating that medical care must be provided in a just manner, we are pointing out that the interests of third parties must be kept in mind. Considerations of justice therefore require that the health care professional take into account how care decisions concerning a patient may affect other persons adversely.

The demand of justice requires in the case of Mrs. Castle that the health care team take into consideration the burdens that their proposed patient management and therapy plans would impose upon other persons. In this case, as the family explained its difficulty, the health care team came to realize and accept that it would be excessively burdensome for the son and daughter-in-law to manage his mother at home. This was not a happy decision. Both the family and the health care team wanted the best for Mrs.Castle. And they recognized that choosing to institutionalize Mrs. Castle would be to her detriment. Yet they also realized that the moral obligations that the son and daughter-in-law had towards their children, particularly their teenaged daughter, and to each other prevented them from caring for Mrs. Castle at home.

How far, though, does this moral obligation to the family extend? Suppose that the son and daughter-in-law were quite willing to take Mrs. Castle back into their home, even knowing that her condition would now require even more time, attention, and energy than ever before. And suppose that the health care team believes that this would be best for Mrs. Castle, but also believes that this could be very harmful to the family. There is already stress between the couple, which exacerbates and is exacerbated by the trouble with the teenaged daughter. Given that Mrs. Castle is their patient, not her family, do they have a moral obligation to recommend to the family that they place her in a nursing home rather than take her back into the house?

Our belief is that if the health care professional thinks that the family is seriously underestimating the difficulty and/or cost to them of the proposed patient care, and the health care professional believes there is a clear potential for significant harm to the family as a result of this underestimation, there is a moral obligation to encourage the family to reconsider.

Our position here may be influenced by our family-oriented approach to medicine, but two reasons can be given for accepting this conclusion. First, it is likely that if the proposed treatment plan actually proved harmful to the family, harm would in turn influence patient care for the worse. Resentment may build toward the elderly patient on the part of overburdened family members. Hence, what had once looked like an ideal patient care setting may transform into one which is actually detrimental. Second, the health care professional has an obligation to avoid serious harm to innocent third parties, including the family.

So far we have considered cases where the harm to the family is relatively clear and significant. What happens, however, when the potential harm is vague or not clearly serious? Consider the following example, where the burden of home care would seem to be relatively light, but the family member does not want to take the patient back into the house after a brief hospitalization.

The Case of Mr. Stern

> Mr. Stern suffers from an insulinoma which originated in the pancreas. Intermittently, the tumor excretes excess insulin and Mr. Stern lapses into a coma from hypoglycemia

and requires hospitalization. During his most recent admission, his wife informed the medical staff that she could no longer care for Mr. Stern at home. Frustrated, he told the attending physician the following:

"I want to go home, but my wife doesn't want me. Look, I'm dying. I know that. I have spent more time in the hospital these past few months than I care to think about. The cancer is all over. It started in the pancreas, but has spread and spread. There's nothing they can do about it.

"My luck—I get some rare disease that bottoms me out and I go into a coma—no warning. They pump me full of sugar and I come right back, but it's got her scared, my wife. Whenever she finds me, she says she doesn't know if it's just another attack or if I'm dead.

"What difference does it make? I'm damned near dead anyway, but she can't accept that.

"It's my house! I paid for it, put my sweat into it! It's my right to die there! She's my wife—'for better or worse, sickness and health' and all that—right? *Is it too much to ask?* I don't need much. Between these attacks, I'm fine, I can take care of myself. I don't need to be here in the hospital and you won't do anything that will make any difference.

"I just need somebody to call the ambulance, or the undertaker . . ."

As Mr. Stern himself has put it, the question here is, how much is "too much" to ask? ·

We have argued that the health care professional has a moral obligation to encourage a family not to take on overly burdensome care obligations. There is a moral obligation, however, to encourage the family to take on care obligations which would be beneficial to the patient and not terribly burdensome to the family.

In the case of Mr. Stern, the burden which Mrs. Stern feels is overwhelmingly of a psychological nature. Constructive counseling, designed to help Mrs. Stern deal with her fears and to face her husband's impending death, could improve both Mr. Stern's final weeks *and* Mrs. Stern's mental health during this period and following her husband's death. The health care team would be doing right in encouraging Mrs. Stern to be counseled in these matters.

Permutations

1. We considered cases where the proposed burden upon the family was either quite heavy or at least perceived as quite heavy. Suppose, however, that the younger Mr. and Mrs. Castle do not want to take his mother into the home because they have planned an extended vacation. What should the health care professionals do?

Some of us expect more from family bonds than others. One who expects a great deal would find the Castles' choice morally offensive. On the other hand, someone who expects very little from family relationships would not be upset by their decision. We suspect that most health care professionals, even if not surprised by their decision, would find it morally unappealing.

While we might find such a decision morally unappealing, the health care professional can not *force* the son to care for his mother (though we could force a father to care for his minor children). One may admonish, cajole, and criticize, but one cannot appeal to legal pressure.

2. Suppose Mrs. Jones lives with her daughter, who takes care of her. A paraplegic, Mrs. Jones is now developing decubiti ulcers which, in her physician's opinion, ought to be managed in a nursing home. Her daughter is unable to provide the kind of therapy which will resolve the ulcers.

    However, the physician also knows that Mrs. Jones' daughter quit her job several years ago in order to move into her mother's apartment and take care of her on a full-time basis. Earning no income herself, and with no real job skills, the daughter has become dependent upon Mrs. Jones' social security check, which supports both of them.

    Should the physician have Mrs. Jones placed in a nursing home, knowing that doing so will put the daughter out in the street with nowhere to go?

In such a case, the daughter will sooner or later have to return to life on her own. In a sense, though, her mother owes her something. For that reason, one may feel it appropriate, if the mother's health permits, to plan a transition period with the daughter. The time period should be clear, with a definite termination. This way, the daughter may be helped along into a more independent life without seriously harming the health of the mother.

Annotated Bibliography

Christie RJ, and Hoffmaster B. *Ethical Issues in Family Medicine,* New York: Oxford University Press,1986.
This is one of the few texts which comes to grips with the ethical difficulties of the physician's relationship with the family through the patient. They persuasively argue that prevalent discussion of autonomy and the physician's obligations to the patient are oversimplified.

References

Christie RJ, and Hoffmaster B. *Ethical Issues in Family Medicine,* New York: Oxford University Press,1986.

CHAPTER 4

The Health Care Team

The Case of Mr. Davis

Mr. Davis was a favorite among the nursing staff at the nursing home. He was always dressed in cardigan sweaters and a tie, strolling through the home with cheery salutations and small talk. His gait was steadied by a twisted briar cane, but his faculties remained pleasantly adled, probably from the years of making rounds at the local pubs. In contrast, the widowed Mrs. Rose was rather stern and prim in her appearance, tending towards dark, matronly clothing. Her dementia was masked largely by her rigid demeanor and withering tongue.

In recent months, and to the bemusement of the staff, Mrs. Rose and Mr. Davis had developed something more than a platonic relationship. The nurses clearly understood the meaning of Mrs. Rose's glare whenever she closed the door to her room behind Mr. Davis, and they took pains to protect this unlikely relationship.

When Mr. Davis suffered a fall and broken hip, the dementia and ataxic gait weighed strongly against his rehabilitation potential. The primary physician, at the recommendation of the orthopedic surgeon, opted for a simple procedure and prolonged bedrest. The nursing staff, however, felt that more extensive surgery involving a hip replacement was appropriate, even though it involved a higher risk. Such a procedure would have a much shorter recovery period and lead to a greater chance for advancement of mobility, both of which they felt were important to Mr. Davis' lifestyle in the nursing home. They were sure that the physicians were overlooking the human side of Mr. Davis.

The nurses enjoined the social worker who had established the closest rapport with Mr. Davis' son to intervene. They took it upon themselves to break their confidence concerning the surreptitious relationship and present their views of the proposed surgery. The son agreed and sought a second opinion from a different physician, who agreed to perform the hip replacement at another hospital.

The procedure went well, much to everyone's relief, and Mr. Davis returned to his room after two weeks. During his convalescence, Mrs. Rose would push Mr. Davis around in his wheelchair until, in time, he became more secure with his walker.

The staff was ecstatic, but their relationship with the primary physician was soured for some time to come. Feeling that his relationship with the family had been undermined and that he had been made to look inept in the eyes of the surgeon, the physician wrote a letter to the chief of nursing accusing the head nurse of insubordination. On subsequent visits to the floor, he withdrew from the nursing staff and was unwilling to discuss patient problems or prognoses with the staff.

Discussion

Three things, in combination, have led to the increasing use of the team approach to health care for the elderly. The first is the vast expansion of medical knowledge and technology which has promoted increased specialization within health care disciplines. Second, as an identifiable segment of the population, the elderly suffer from a greater number of medical illnesses or conditions per capita than other groups. Numerous health care providers from different specialties are involved, often simultaneously, in their care. The coordination of services has been seen as a mechanism to improve the efficiency of health care delivery through decreased redundancy and the exchange and discussion of information from a variety of specialty backgrounds.

The proper use of the team approach can also improve the *ethical* quality of patient care. Our goal in this chapter is to explore some of the ethically distinctive features of health care professionals working together as a team. This approach underlies the decision-making process discussed in Part II.

4.1 Team Responsibility

The traditional understanding of ethical responsibility in the delivery of health care regards the physician as the professional who carries both moral authority and moral responsibility. This approach is founded on the traditional hierarchy of professionals in the acute hospital and, to some degree, from the physician as the CEO of his private office practice. In these settings, other health care workers are clearly subordinates who carry out the will of the physician. However, in the complex, multi-dimensional setting of chronic care, the physician grows increasingly reliant on the skills and knowledge of other professionals. This forces us to reassess such views of moral authority and responsibility and to regard them as no longer appropriate. Moral responsibility and authority is no longer the purview of the physician alone, but the *team* itself is a moral agent with the physician as its titular head.

One key feature of the team approach is that it recognizes that different health care workers have valuable contributions to make in deciding on approaches to care. But now, as team members, it becomes their moral responsibility to share such information or insights. Not to do so is to lessen the quality of care of the patient. Thus, the principles of autonomy and beneficence extend to all members of the team. The team, however, is not just an assortment of individuals who happen to be caring for the same patient. This is different from saying that the physician is responsible as a physician, and the nurse as a nurse, and the social worker as a social worker, etc. What we are suggesting, as has been well argued by Thomasma (1981), is that the *team* as a *unit* bears moral responsibility. The team represents the coordinated efforts of all its members as a single entity. Responsibility is shared jointly, as is credit or blame.

In concert with these changes in approach, there has been an extension of liability such that the team members as well as the physician are often named in lawsuits concerning issues of malpractice. The institution, as employer, is also increasingly involved in such cases, and can therefore be seen as an important influence on team decision making.

4.2 Ethical Decision Making in the Team

If the team has such moral responsibility as an agent, then in some sense each individual member of the team can be morally praiseworthy or blameworthy on account of what the team as a whole decides and does. Developing a group decision-making process whereby each member of the team has the opportunity to play a *meaningful* role in making ethical decisions is, however, more difficult than one might think. If the team acts contrary to the moral convictions of one of its members, then that member becomes in his or her mind, by extension, morally guilty of some act. The understandable attempt to avoid such guilt feelings can easily lead to alienation from the rest of the team and breakdown of the benefits which were to accrue from the team approach to care.

Thomasma (1981) argues that there are five requisites for constructive decision making in the team setting. The first three deal with knowledge and attitudes, and the remainder with practice skills. First, the health care team must share a common moral vocabulary. If the team members are not using words in the same way and with the same implications, then they are not communicating effectively and thereby undermine the validity of the moral consensus. Second, the team must, as a whole, have some training and experience in the articulation of moral feelings and beliefs. Third, the team, through education, must learn to distinguish moral values from other sorts of values, and must also learn of the plurality of moral values which surrounds us. An appreciation of the possible differences in ethical values among the team members (and between the team and the patient) can help foster consensus.

Fourth, the team, through experience, must develop a sense of what might count as a moral issue. Then, the team's decision-making process should be structured in such a way that potential ethical difficulties are brought to light and considered. Fifth and finally, each of the team members must employ (and participate in) the same decision-making process. If all members are working with the same sorts of equations, it is far more likely that they will reach a mutually tolerable consensus. This requires that protocols for both the content and timeliness for patient review be established for the delineation of treatment plans, and that specific steps be defined in coming to agreement in limiting these plans. (Limited treatment plans are discussed in chapter 7.) Use of these protocols should therefore effectively minimize feelings of alienation since each team member will more easily understand the reasoning and process of decision making which motivates and directs the rest of the team in its decisions.

Occasionally, there will be a team member who has serious moral disagreements with many of the team's decisions. Moral differences among the team members are inevitable, whether brought to light or not. These differences, left unacknowledged and undiscussed, will cause friction and dissent which not only make the workplace unpleasant but which may actually harm the patient's interests. The decision-making process which we recommend will highlight such differences and open up three possible resolutions. First, if the dispute is neither serious nor chronic, the dissenting member may choose to go along with the rest of the team for the sake of harmony. If, however, the difference is of a more serious nature, the team member should be allowed to withdraw from participation in the case in question and to record his or her dissent. Finally, if the ethical decision-making process reveals chronic and significant ethical disagreements between a member of the team and the rest of the team, the individual may recognize the nature of the disagreement and may choose to transfer to a different team rather than face frequent ethical discord and alienation.

Mr. Davis' case illustrates what can happen when a health care team lacks an open and effective decision-making process for ethically laden choices. Because of the way in which the decision was made, the ethical implications of the treatment decision never came to light, much less were resolved by the team. A more thoughtful process, which gave voice to the various concerns of the staff, would have brought the value-laden nature of the alternatives into the open.

4.3 Effective Communication

We have so far emphasized that the team must be effective in its communication of ethical values, beliefs, and the like. It is also true that the team, if it is to operate effectively, must communicate patient care information with each other. A team works best when the various members all know what the game strategy is. Without knowledge of the overall strategy, individual team members will not always be able to help or warn other team members of unseen or unforeseen difficulties that might hamper patient care. Furthermore, if members of the team feel that their voices have not been heard or that a case has been handled unjustly, resentment will build, destroying the working integrity of the team.

In order to foster effective communication, there should be certain agreed upon procedures or mechanisms for bringing to light and addressing ethical values in patient care.

First, the team needs to negotiate general care policies and procedures with the institutional administration. For example, the team should establish policies (or affirm existing policies) outlining institutional policies towards advance directives, do-not-treat, do-not-transfer and do-not-resuscitate orders. Included in such policies should be set procedures for:

- Filing such orders, including such seemingly mundane concerns as what sorts of forms ought to be used and what information they must register.
- An understanding of when the institutional administration needs to be involved, including referral to legal counsel.
- An understanding of under what circumstances the Institutional Ethics Committee *must* be involved.
- An understanding of when advice *can* be sought from the Institutional Ethics Committee.

Second, the team itself must establish a discussion process which ensures consideration of ethical concerns.

- Will there be a set meeting schedule (e.g., once a week)?
- Who will function as the chair of the meeting?
- Will discussion be round robin, requiring some word from each involved team member? Or will it be more of an ad hoc discussion?

Third, since the team as a whole is responsible for patient care decisions, the team must keep a written record of its decision making. Hence, there needs to be a recording secretary who:

- Notes the substance of the discussion and makes the appropriate entries in the patient's chart.
- Makes the appropriate or required notification to the administration or Institutional Ethics Committee.

Fourth, the team must decide how and under what circumstances it will deal with the patient's family.

- What sort of consultation with the family is required under what sorts of circumstances?
- Who will act as a liaison between the team and the family, if necessary?

Fifth, who will decide the agenda for the team meeting? Will the team review all cases, even if it touches upon some only briefly? Or will only certain cases be discussed at any one meeting? Who decides which cases?

Many of these may seem rather mundane concerns, but they can be quite important issues. Having such established policies and procedures for decision making encourages the consideration of the many ethical dimensions which a case might have. Furthermore, if the team has such policies and procedures and keeps a record of its discussion and decision making, families and patients are less likely to quarrel with patient care or patient care decisions. Finally, if a lawsuit does develop, the documentation of the team's decision-making process can demonstrate that ethical considerations did play a role, that there was discussion, and that patient care decisions were neither haphazard nor heartless. This can protect both the team and the institution.

4.4 Issues of Confidentiality

While the team approach can enhance patient care, it also requires reconsideration of traditional conceptions of physician-patient confidentiality. If the team is truly to operate as a *team*, it is necessary for the various team members, including the physician, to be able to share patient information which would traditionally be considered confidential. The question, then, is how best to move from a relationship of strict physician-patient confidentiality to one in which patient information may be shared among the various members of the team.

Patient education is the key to consent. If the professional can promote an understanding of the value of the team approach to health care, the patient will most likely agree to an expansion of the circle of confidentiality. As noted in chapter 2, however, it need not be necessary for the patient to agree that the physician share *all* patient information. If the patient is incompetent, the physician has a moral obligation to reach an agreement with the appropriate family or designated guardian in the same manner.

An important corollary is that as the domain of those with access to information increases, so does the number of persons who are obligated to preserve patient confidentiality. Many of the members of the health care team in addition to the physician will already be under a professional obligation to respect patient confidentiality. The duty to keep patient information confidential, however, ought to be emphasized to all team members. The constructiveness of the health care provider-patient relationship is grounded in trust, and that trust must not be jeopardized by the careless divulgence of sensitive information to persons outside of the team.

4.5 The Team versus the System

We have discussed ways in which the sharing of medical and patient knowledge among the team members can improve patient care. One must not forget, however, that the health care team operates within an institution which is but a part of a highly fragmented and increasingly regulated health care system. In particular, the team may have to act as an advocate for the patient. Let us consider two ways in which this might happen.

Health care resources, in certain circumstances, are limited. This does not entail everyone receiving an equally small share, however. Beds in ICUs or rehabilitative institutions, for example, will be in short supply. It will be morally incumbent upon the health care team when they believe they have a patient who deserves the benefits of these services to act as advocates for their patient to increase his or her chances of getting that precious space.

A second way in which the team may be called upon to advocate for their patients regards finances. The vast majority of elderly patients have inadequate health insurance to cover the enormous expenses of long term care. Furthermore, most Medicaid systems require that elderly persons pay for health care costs out of their own resources until they are themselves impoverished. Although it would be morally wrong to falsify or fabricate documents or diagnoses, the health care team does have a moral obligation to make as much legitimate use of the reimbursement systems as possible on behalf of the patient.

4.6 Case Revisited

The Davis case is an illustration of the health care team in moral (and medical) disarray. It seems evident that there was no set mechanism for the allied health professionals to bring their concerns before the attending physician. Even informal discussion between the physician and other team members seems to have been sadly absent. This led to the nurses approaching the patient's family behind the back of the physician. The physician took this both as a breach of trust and as an insult to his professional competence; he regarded their behavior as insubordination. And as matters went, the dynamics of the health care team continued to deteriorate.

If there had been a team decision procedure accepted by all members there would have been no need for this divisiveness. The concerns of each member of the team, including the physician, could have been brought into a candid discussion. If the physician continued to have very strong reservations, the matter (according to team policy) could have been brought before the responsible family members with both viewpoints presented and explained. If the treatment decision is reached through mutually accepted team decision procedures, it should be a mutually acceptable decision, even if not all team members endorse the recommendation without reservation.

It has long been understood that a significant part of the health care professional's ability to heal rests in the patient's confidence in the practitioner. When the patient or family is presented with a team that is acrimoniously divided amongst itself and in decisional disarray, that confidence is eroded. It is the moral responsibility of the health care team as the provider of health care to ensure that it can effectively deal with the ethical complexion of health care delivery *as a team*.

4.7 Conclusion

We have argued that the delivery of health care by a team, as is particularly appropriate for the sorts of problems frequently faced by elderly patients, is ethically different from the traditional delivery of health care with the physician as the sole medical authority. The ethical challenge is for the team to develop the skills and procedures that encourage coherent and satisfactory ethical decision making as a team.

Permutations

1. Suppose that in Mr. Davis' case the physician agreed with the nurses about the proper surgical therapy, but that there was no family to consult. Since Mr. Davis is incompetent and there is no dissent, can they just go ahead and do the surgery?

Surgical procedures require informed consent except under special circumstances which require immediate action, such as emergency conditions. Since Mr. Davis is evidently incompetent, he cannot give informed consent. Hence, the responsibility for decision making typically falls upon the attending physician. But the authority of the attending physician is intended only as a temporary measure for the needs of such special conditions as emergencies. It is expected that the health care team will petition the courts for a hearing on Mr. Davis' competence and if found legally incompetent, then a legal guardian will be appointed by the court. Only once this is done, and a legally appointed guardian exists, should any non-emergency surgery (or other medical procedures requiring consent) be done.

2. Suppose that, as the case happened, there was dissent within the team. Suppose further that the family is either indecisive or non-existent. What should then be done?

We suggest that in this kind of scenario appeal to the Institutional Ethics Committee would be appropriate. The team dissent ought to be dealt with as much as possible prior to appeal to the courts.

3. Suppose that though the team was unanimously agreed, the family was strongly opposed to the more drastic surgical procedure.

The family never has absolute decision-making authority over a patient, even when the patient is incompetent. The appropriate first step would be a meeting with the family in an attempt to resolve differences. The second step would be appeal to the institutional ethics committee. Failing resolution, appeal to the courts would be appropriate.

Annotated Bibliography

Very little has been written on the ethical complexity of the team approach to health care delivery. The article relating most directly with the ethics of team care is Thomasma's. For a more general, though useful, discussion of team dynamics see the chapter authored by Maguire.

Maguire GH. "The Team Approach In Action," Chapter 18 of *Care of the Elderly: A Health Team Approach,* (edited by GH Maguire) Boston: Little, Brown and Co., 1985.
An excellent not written with ethics in mind, this is a helpful analysis of why the team care approach can be beneficial for elderly patients.

Thomasma DC. "Moral Education in Interdisciplinary Teams," *Prospectus for Change* 6:1–4 (1981).
An excellent analysis of team decision making in the health professions. Includes practical suggestions on how to promote effective team decision making.

References

Thomasma DC. "Moral Education in Interdisciplinary Teams," *Prospectus for Change* 6:1–4 (1981).

CHAPTER 5

The Institutional Ethics Committee

The Case of Mr. Harrison

Mr. Harrison was a 72-year-old gentleman who had been living in a boarding home since his wife died in the early 1980s. He was brought to the emergency room by his landlady because of severe depression accompanied by weight loss and diarrhea, and admitted to the psychiatric service. The original diagnostic evaluation concluded that the diarrhea was a chronic symptom of a "dumping syndrome" attendant to a gastric resection done several years ago for peptic ulcers; the more recent onset of weight loss was a manifestation of his depression and anorexia. The diarrhea persisted despite treatment and improvement of the affective symptoms, however, so further studies were ordered. These revealed the true underlying cause of Mr. Harrison's illness: adenocarcinoma of the rectum with liver metastases.

He was evaluated by a surgical oncologist who recommended a resection of the tumor and a permanent colostomy in order to obviate future obstruction, relieve him of the diarrhea and allow him to regain his nutritional balance. Mr. Harrison was informed of his diagnosis and approached by the surgeons for consent to the proposed procedure, to which he agreed. When the anesthesiologist came for a pre-operative assessment, Mr. Harrison denied any knowledge of his cancer and was quite upset that no one had discussed this with him previously!

The psychiatrist was called and explained that Mr. Harrison suffered from a moderate degree of dementia which primarily affected his memory. Through the course of their discussion, the doubts of Mr. Harrison's competence for informed consent became increasingly tangible. The anesthesiologist was unwilling to accept the patient for surgery. The psychiatrist was also concerned that the trauma of anesthesia and changes in his body image could exacerbate his dementia and depression, having significant consequences on the quality of his remaining life—which, with liver metastases, was not likely to be long.

Meanwhile, the geriatric consultation team had also been asked by the surgeon to see this patient for medical clearance. The geriatrician reviewed the case and felt that, although his nutritional parameters increased the operative risks, these would not likely improve with time and the benefits held sway. Her recommendations were in accord with the surgeon, but on discussing the various options with Mr. Harrison, she also found him unaware of this diagnosis. She presented the facts again and Mr. Harrison concluded that surgery was the appropriate course. Thus, the geriatrician felt that he was capable of consent since when given the circumstances, he was consistent in his decisions.

In the geriatric consultation team meeting, it became apparent that the other members were not supportive of the decision for surgery. The nurse felt that the marked memory impairment rendered him incapable of learning the self-care skills necessary for management of the colostomy, and that he had already accommodated to donning and wearing diapers. The social worker added that if he could not tend to his colostomy independently, the boarding home would not likely allow him back, and therefore he would require nursing home placement prematurely. As his disease progressed, he would need to make a second move to a higher level facility, a disruptive and potentially avoidable consequence if the surgery were not done at this time.

A team meeting was convened. It became clear that there was no consensus on which course of action to recommend nor on Mr. Harrison's competency, or who should ultimately take responsibility for his care.

Discussion

Hospital ethics committees have their origin in 1960 when long term dialysis became medically possible. The extremely small number of dialysis machines combined with the large number of potential candidates for long term dialysis made it necessary to decide who would and who would not receive dialysis. (Ross JW 1986). Not wanting to make these decisions alone, the physicians involved organized committees composed of physicians, other health professionals, and lay persons. Though the shortage of dialysis machines was eventually resolved, other ethically difficult challenges have emerged. For example, the court judgment in the Karen Ann Quinlan case recommended that hospital ethics committees (then called "prognosis committees") be formed to consider cases involving the termination of life-support technology for irreversibly comatose patients. More recently, attention has been focused upon infant care review committees. In response to these ethically difficult situations, more and more health care facilities have established institutional ethics committees (IEC). The JCAHO has stipulated that all hospitals should have IECs by 1988. And the trend is being joined by long-term care institutions. (Ross JW 1986.)

This chapter is not intended to offer guidelines on how to form IECs, or on who should sit on such committees, or how many members the committee should have. There are many other sources which provide thorough discussion of such matters. (See the annotated bibliography at the end of this chapter for such references.) What we wish to explore is how and why the IEC can be particularly useful for the health care professional caring for elderly patients.

There are several reasons why the professional caring for elderly patients may find it useful to turn to an IEC.

- Care of elderly patients, particularly those in long term care institutions, is frequently characterized by the *team approach*. This requires the team to be able to make ethical decisions *as a team*, something which is not always easy.
- Care of the ill elderly frequently raises questions concerning institutional policies. Under what sorts of circumstances is it permissible to limit treatment, including life-sustaining treatment? What sorts of procedures must be followed in deciding to withhold or

withdraw treatment from a patient? Chronic illness also frequently poses a choice between numerous alternatives, increasing the possibility of disagreement between providers and patient or between team members.

- Family can play a significant but often ethically ambiguous role. The offspring of elderly patients are themselves adults and are often called upon or insist upon taking a role in decision making. The financial interests of the family as a whole may be at issue, giving rise to conflict of interest between patient and family. This raises questions of confidentiality, authority, and conflict of interest, making medical decision making quite complicated.

- Though we should not accept the terrible stereotype that all elderly suffer from dementia, we must admit that the incidence of dementia is significantly higher among the elderly. When encountered, dementia (and also *marginal competence*) greatly complicates decision-making procedures.

The key here is to learn how to make use of the IEC to facilitate the delivery of high ethical quality care. For the purposes of discussion, we shall point out three kinds of assistance that can be sought from an IEC.

5.1 Education in Ethical Decision Making

As discussed in the preceding chapter, the team approach to providing health care for the elderly requires that the team be able to engage constructively in ethical decision making. This entails that the team must share a moral vocabulary as well as an effective and ethically sensitive decision-making procedure. There must be a mutual understanding as to the meaning of specific terms and agreement on a framework of ethical theory. Additionally, the team must develop a mechanism to assure that all ethically relevant issues are discussed at the meetings so that important decisions are not inadvertently left to a few members. None of these conditions are likely to be met by lucky happenstance. Rather, they must be reached through education and practice.

The IEC can be a useful source of skill and expertise in these matters, making arrangements for seminars for the health care team taught by committee members or recommending someone outside of the committee who is trained in ethics. This might be a member of the philosophy department of a nearby university or medical school who specializes in ethics or medical ethics. Many medical schools, hospitals, and nursing homes are now retaining such persons on a part-time basis to assist in matters such as this.

The majority of health care is provided in ambulatory care settings and in smaller nursing homes which are not likely to be able to support their own IECs. In these instances, the local medical society may provide a committee structure, with representation from related health care professions, to act as a resource for physicians in the community faced with ethical dilemmas. The probability that members from hospital and nursing home ethics committees will also participate provides a unique opportunity for a broader perspective to be brought to the decision-making process across all settings of care.

5.2 Clarification of Institutional Policy

It can frequently happen that the health care professional is not sure of institutional policies affecting patient care. Two different, but closely related, sorts of questions arise. First, what sorts of practices are permitted by the institution? For example, the health care professional may want to know what the institutional policies are concerning an incompetent patient in the face of family disagreement. Also unclear could be institutional policies involving the withdrawal of nutrition and hydration, discontinuance of ventilator support, etc. For obvious reasons, it is important that the professional *know* what is and is not permitted by the institution where the patient is located.

It is not enough, however, only to know what is or is not permitted. One must also know the accepted or required procedures for reaching such treatment (or non-treatment) decisions. This involves questions of:

- Authority—Who has the authority to make decisions? The competent patient? The physician? The family? The health care team? Or some combination of them? Does the institution have the right to impose certain sorts of decisions? Most likely, authority will rest in some combination of the parties, and an IEC can help to clarify the various roles these parties may play in decision making.
- Procedure—Is there a specific process through which this decision must be reached? Can it be decided by a

discussion between family and patient? Must it involve review by the IEC? Must the administration be consulted or notified? Even if the IEC does not play a role in the decision making of a specific case, it can offer helpful information on the procedural format that these very important decisions must follow.

When there is any confusion in these matters, the health care professional should approach the IEC for clarification.

Finally, when the health care professional encounters ethically controversial situations which have not been addressed, or where an institutional policy seems mistaken or objectionable, the professional should approach the IEC about developing or altering institutional policy.

5.3 Consultation

A third way in which the health care professional may find the IEC of assistance is through consultation on specific cases. It should be clarified at this point that the IEC is not the decision-making body nor the final arbiter; rather, its role is that of a facilitator and resource of information and procedural guidelines. Therefore, the role is very much consultative and educational. There are at least three situations which might make it appropriate to seek an IEC review.

The first is dissension. There are a number of ways in which dissension may appear during a decision-making process. There may be dissension between the team and the family. There may be dissension within the team. The team may be in disagreement with other professional opinions. And the team, in conjunction with the patient or family, may be in disagreement with the institutional administration. For the good of the particular patient involved, the good of future patients, team members, and the institution, such dissension must be dealt with in an ethically just manner. This is best done by approaching the IEC and appealing to it as an impartial but well-informed third party to provide a forum for discussion as well as constructive suggestions on how to reach an acceptable decision. Many of these presumed disputes are really motivated by a sense that someone's position is not heard or is not being considered fairly, and the involvement of an impartial IEC can serve to defuse this kind of conflict and assist the parties in reaching their own agreement.

The second reason for seeking IEC case consultation is that it might be institutional policy to require IEC review of certain kinds of cases. For example, some institutions require IEC review of all life-threatening decisions concerning incompetent patients, even where there is no dissension within or between the health care team and the family or guardian to ensure that those who are unable to speak for themselves have their interests adequately safeguarded. Thus, for instance, some institutions may require IEC review of any decision to withhold CPR, nutrition and hydration, or other life-sustaining therapy for an incompetent patient.

Third, the health care professional may find it useful to approach the IEC for guidelines concerning processes of legal adjudication. Since many of these cases may require guardianship, it is important for the health care team to help the family choose a responsible person, or to request oversight through the state office on aging. Second, the team should establish a recommended course of action to be presented to the court for approval. A designated physician will also be needed to testify at the proceedings. Finally, the decision will need to be made as to whether the case should be presented by the hospital counsel, a private attorney or representation sought through adult protective services.

5.4 The Ethical Standing of IEC Statements

Much of the resistance to IECs on the part of health care professionals has been based upon two beliefs. The first objection is that an IEC interferes with the privacy of the provider-patient relationship. The second objection is that the IEC can bind the physician against his or her will. Let us consider each of these in turn.

Objecting to IECs on the grounds that they violate the privacy of the provider-patient relationship ignores the fact that health care is delivered in the context of society, even if the provider-patient encounter takes place in the privacy of the physician's office. For instance, physicians are not permitted to practice substandard medicine or prescribe harmful treatments. Further, they are required to report to public health authorities information on instances of certain dangerous and communicable diseases. These serve merely as examples of the fact that societal interests already play a morally legitimate role in the provider-patient relationship. And when health care is delivered in the setting of a specific institution, it is not unreasonable for the institution to take an interest in the quality of care delivered, including the ethical quality of that care. Finally, it is recognized as good medical practice to seek a second opinion when a particular problem extends beyond the area of one's own expertise. Referral to an IEC is in principle quite similar to other sorts of consultations.

As with other forms of consultations, the members of the IEC can only perform their task by being informed of the details of the cases. However, this information is recognized as being of both a personal and sensitive nature and should be treated in a most confidential manner.

The second objection is based on the concern that the counsel of the IEC establishes a binding standard of care. This issue has two components. To begin with, it is true that the IEC is often the responsible administrative mechanism for the development of institutional policies and procedures in this area, and that these decisions are binding upon the health care professional. On the other hand, the rationale behind IECs is to offer assistance to health professionals and patients in sorting out the ethical complexities of the case in question. Inasmuch as the IEC is staffed by persons experienced in these matters and well-versed in ethics, their advice should not be taken lightly. However, the counsel offered in specific cases should be regarded as just that, counsel. Only the court holds final authority.

5.5 Case Revisited

The decisional dilemmas presented in the case of Mr. Harrison are not uncommon. All too often there is no clear direction, yet neither action nor inaction are without consequences. The importance of this case is not so much the resolution as the process by which the conclusion was reached. The success of the institutional ethics committee is an example of the benefits of an outside facilitator experienced in interdisciplinary negotiation and assistance in directing the professionals to an acceptable outcome.

The geriatric consultant had sensed disagreement within her own team as well as among the others involved, and recommended an impartial arbitration. The facts of the case were presented by the psychiatrist and the geriatrician to an interdisciplinary panel comprised of three members of the institutional ethics committee.* They were the first to recognize that no one was actually in charge. Mr. Harrison had been admitted to the psychiatric service but now had a medical-surgical problem. All the physicians were acting as consultants and there was no appropriate primary care practitioner to weigh the various and conflicting opinions. They also recommended that he be referred to adult protective services for evaluation of competency as his condition was likely to require the help of a guardian within the near future. Only if surgery was to be pursued should an expedited guardianship be sought with the assistance of the hospital's administration. The patient was therefore transferred to the family medicine service.

The family physician reviewed the consultations and interviewed Mr. Harrison who, although again quite perturbed when told of his cancer, elected to undergo surgery. The administration was asked to facilitate guardianship proceedings. They determined that Mr. Harrison's judgment was consistent, and so should be respected, but that he was incompetent to sign consent due to his marked memory disturbance. The judge brought him under the protection of the court and assigned responsibility for his care to the state office on aging with permission to allow surgery.

Mr. Harrison fared better than we had reason to hope. His landlady at the boarding home was willing to learn colostomy care and he returned after an uneventful post-operative course. He is now followed by the family physician as an outpatient with the help of the hospital's home care nursing and social work staff.

5.6 Conclusion

Providing health care for the elderly can be ethically complex. Increased incidences of dependency, dementia of varying degrees, chronic illnesses, and team-provided care all contribute to the difficulty in recognizing all the ethically significant features of case management. The health care professional should look upon the IEC not as an intrusive enemy but as a committee of skilled persons who can act as a resource in assisting the professional, the patient, and family in reaching ethically acceptable decisions.

*The IEC in large institutions is often comprised of several representatives from all the clinical departments. This becomes an unwieldy group for readily available consultation, so a panel of three members drawn at random is chosen for each case.

Permutations

> 1. What if Mr. Harrison was clearly demented and not competent to participate in the decision-making process?

Although the outcome may have been different, there would still have been the imperative to establish a responsible voice for both the patient and the medical-surgical staff. In fact, the recommendations of the IEC would not have been affected.

> 2. What if the illness were not life-threatening?

The IEC would not need to become involved. The fact that Mr. Harrison had recovered from the symptoms which prompted hospitalization would lead us to recommend that he be discharged to a primary care physician and referred to adult protective services (APS) for evaluation. The discharge summary should report the APS referral and reflect the various opinions and lack of consensus in treatment of the illness, leaving resolution to the new physician. No further action needs to be taken toward guardianship unless the seriousness of the illness changes. This does not preclude a family member from seeking guardianship through a private attorney. Assignment of a durable power of attorney, however, would not be appropriate.

Annotated Bibliography

Cranford RE, and Doudera AE (eds.). *Institutional Ethics Committees and Health Care Decision Making.* Ann Arbor: Health Administration Press, 1984.
This volume contains the proceedings of a national conference on institutional ethics committees, helpful information on several existing ethics committees, and sample policies and guidelines.
Minnesota Medical Association, Committee on Ethics and Medical-Legal Affairs. "Institutional Ethics Committees," *Minnesota Medicine* 68:607-12 (1985).
Suggested guidelines for the institution of ethics committees.
Ross JW. *Handbook for Hospital Ethics Committees.* Chicago: American Hospital Publishing, 1986.

This is an excellent handbook on the history and scope of ethics committees and how to institute one. The best general introduction to institutional ethics committees.

Thomasma DC. "Hospital Ethics Committees and Hospital Policy," *QRB* July 1985:204-09.

Thomasma discusses the functions of an IEC as well as pointing out the importance of ethics committees in the hospital setting.

Wolf SM. "Ethics Committees in the Courts," *Hastings Center Report,* Special Supplement, June 1986, pp. 12-15.

Wolf analyzes how courts have regarded recommendations made by IECs. While some courts have chosen to ignore IEC recommendations, others have used IEC recommendations as admissible evidence. Wolf argues that courts should, in some cases, make use of the recommendations of the IEC in making and structuring their decisions.

References

Ross JW. *Handbook for Hospital Ethics Committees.* Chicago: American Hospital Publishing, 1986.

CHAPTER 6

Research and the Elderly

The Case of Dr. Ratzan

In the late 1970s, Dr. Ratzan was interested in doing research in nursing homes. The setting provided a captive audience and the field of geriatric medicine was in its infancy in this country. He worked half-time in a fine long term care facility, the other half at the local university-affiliated hospital with both the academic talent and manpower from which to draw. A student approached him with a project that, although of marginal interest, was relatively simple in design and likely to produce publishable results with a small population. The home certainly had the potential to gather a sufficient number of subjects.

The medical director was very supportive and provided the time, expertise and direction for an institutional review board to assure compliance with nationally established guidelines. Recommendations for research within the institutional settings were also followed and several additional safeguards were added to match their particular circumstances.

Of the 315 patients in the home, 107 were receiving the medication to be studied. Sixty passed the first screen for competency, but only 24 passed a more thorough second evaluation. This group would be interviewed for the final phase. Unfortunately, the private physicians refused access to 13 of these finalists. And worse, none of the remaining 11 patients would volunteer! Most of those involved seemed concerned about the venepuncture—a not infrequent occurrence—and others did not wish to be bothered. Advice from both peers and family played a strong role. The resistance was widespread; change and knowledge were frightening, indeed!

But despite the setback, the researchers remained undeterred. After all, enlightenment takes time. The mechanisms were in place and there would surely be another opportunity. Oh, and by the way, Dr. Ratzan was right about his study producing publishable results. His experience found its way to print: "The experiment that wasn't: A case report in clinical geriatric research." *Gerontologist* 21:297-302 (1981). It has become a guide, and a warning, to all those who have followed.

Discussion

Medical research, including human experimentation, is an integral part of medicine. We must accept that medical experimentation can be morally good. We might even go so far as to argue that under certain conditions the special obligation of the health care professional can make medical research (including human experimentation) morally obligatory. Nevertheless, research can easily be morally abusive. To avoid that unwanted possibility, therefore, we must ask what ethical principles should guide us in conducting research. And for our purposes in particular, we must ask what special ethical considerations should be kept in mind when experimenting upon elderly subjects. We will begin by reviewing ethical principles appropriate to human research in general, with special reference to *The Belmont Report*. We shall then consider the special concerns which must be considered in using elderly subjects for experimentation.

6.1 Ethical Principles of Research in General

As a result of increasing public concern in the late 1960s over the potential for abuse of human subjects, the federal government established the National Commission for the Protection of Human Subjects of Biomedical and Behavioral Research. This Commission issued its final conclusions in 1978 as a document which became known as *The Belmont Report*. The report emphasized three ethical principles which should be central to conducting human research—respect for persons, beneficence, and justice.

The principle of respect for persons focuses on the autonomy of individuals. This principle is the basis of our moral obligation to seek informed consent prior to medical interventions. Individuals who are competent should be allowed to make their own informed choices about participation or non-participation in medical research. The Commission was especially concerned that those individuals who are incompetent to make such choices by themselves should be protected from abuse. Hence the use of subjects of diminished autonomy must meet even more stringent requirements than the use of competent individuals.

The second principle, beneficence, concerns the health professional's moral obligation to do good, rather than harm, for patients. Since research often poses some risk for the subject, the Commission argues that experiments are ethical only when there is a reasonable balance of benefits over risks. That is, the "risk-benefit ratio" should be substantially on the benefit side. If there is not an acceptable ratio, then the research project should be reformulated or not pursued at all.

Third, the principle of justice requires that the risks of research should be equitably distributed. Prior to the Commission, for example, institutionalized individuals, such as those in nursing homes, psychiatric facilities, and prisons, were enrolled in research projects far out of proportion to their numbers in society at large simply because of their easy availability. This was not equitable, and hence it was not morally just.

In order to assess the ethical acceptability of particular research proposals, the Commission required that all institutions conducting human research involving any government money must have an "Institutional Review Board." This IRB would be responsible for reviewing all research proposals involving human subjects to ensure that the project is in conformity with the three principles discussed above.

The Commission has, on the whole, been a great moral success. Nevertheless, some questions remain unanswered.

First, it is not always clear how the risk-benefit assessment should proceed. Suppose, for example, that a proposed project entails significant risk to the subject and offers little or no therapeutic advantage to the subject. At first glance, this would not be an acceptable research project because of its unfavorable risk-benefit ratio. But suppose further that the information gained could well prove beneficial to persons suffering in the future. Is it ethically proper to ask someone to suffer now, with no prospect of benefit to himself, so that others whom he does not know might benefit in the future? Are there good reasons why a patient should be willing to participate in research? If the research project offers a beneficial therapeutic possibility to the patient involved with an acceptable risk, then it could clearly be in the self-interest of the patient to participate. The more difficult cases, however, are those where there is some risk involved but no therapeutic benefit for the subject. How can we, as health care professionals committed to benefiting and not harming our patients, ask our patients to undergo risk without the hope of any benefit to themselves? This question becomes particularly vexing when dealing with incompetent patients, where proxy consent must be sought. Is it morally acceptable to enroll Alzheimer's patients in research which will not benefit them, though it may benefit future Alzheimer's victims? Can one accept a proxy's consent for such research?

A second concern, expressed by Cassel (1987), is that the Commission has required us to be *over*zealous in protecting vulnerable individuals from abuse. What were intended as protective procedures have become, instead, barriers to important research. The result, she argues, is that many reasonable, important, potentially beneficial, and ethical research projects were never implemented because of overly protective regulations. The consequence has been far less progress in controlling or ameliorating the medical problems which frequently afflict the very segments of the population which we have sought to protect from abuse.

Let us return to our first question for a moment, whether there are good reasons for participating in non-therapeutic research. As posed, the question presupposes that all patients are fundamentally selfish in nature, that they would be unwilling to risk harm to themselves in order to provide benefits for others. This presupposition runs counter to our experience of human nature. Most people are to some extent altruistic. They have a desire to help others in need even at cost to the self. Respect for autonomy, therefore, implies that the health care professional should respect the fact that some patients do have this morally noble desire and that one should not unreasonably frustrate that altruistic desire.

One might also argue that our patients today are the beneficiaries of the risks accepted by others in past research projects. As beneficiaries, therefore, they owe a debt of gratitude to society, a debt that can only be paid by participating in research themselves for the benefit of future patients. This debt of gratitude is surely an "imperfect duty," that is, it is not a duty that we can legitimately *compel* other persons to fulfill. Nevertheless, it would not be morally improper to *encourage* patients to fulfill their debt of gratitude.

For some patients, particularly for those beyond cure, the opportunity to give of themselves for the benefit of others can provide a sense of meaning or purpose for their lives. To exclude them from research simply because it puts them at risk without offering them any commensurable medical benefit would be to deprive them of the possibility of contributing to their community. We should not deprive our patients by unreasonably discouraging participation in research.

6.2 Research with the Elderly

There are many special characteristics which make the elderly, as a group, deserving of special ethical consideration as subjects for research. Our discussion will be divided under two headings: (A) reasons for participation, and (B) reasons for special protection from abuse.

A. Reasons for Participation

Ignoring possible beneficial therapy for the research subject, there are, we believe, stronger moral obligations for the elderly to participate in "non-therapeutic" research than for other age groups. This is for three reasons. To begin with, by being elderly, it is more likely that they have benefited from past research than other members of society. Hence, as their benefit has been great, their debt of gratitude is correspondingly greater. Granted, we should not *force* anyone to show gratitude. Nevertheless, it is morally appropriate to encourage persons to fulfill such obligations.

Second, as persons approach the end of life, the remaining years are more readily balanced with other concerns. This means that many elderly persons (especially the "old-old") simply do not assess risks in the same way as young or middle aged persons. What might be "lost" or suffered is just not the same as it would be in the case of a much younger person, perhaps a child whose life is still ahead or a parent with responsibility for nurturing offspring.

Third, much research, particularly research related to age-specific conditions, can *only* be done effectively with geriatric subjects. For example, substantial progress in treating and preventing Alzheimer's type disease can only be made by research involving Alzheimer's victims, the vast majority of whom are elderly. (The case of Alzheimer's disease and other dementias raises a special issue of consent, which is discussed below. See also Melnick VL, et al., 1984.)

There are many morally acceptable, even morally admirable, reasons why elderly persons might wish to participate in risky research or in research that offers no therapeutic benefit to themselves as individuals. Although we should never compel research participation against a patient's will (except in the special case of incompetent patients who stand to greatly benefit from therapeutic research), we should not deprive the elderly from research participation simply because of their advanced age and increased vulnerability.

B. Reasons for Special Protection

There is nothing about being aged, *per se*, which mandates special moral treatment. An aged person is a moral agent just as any other adult person. Yet there are several conditions which afflict the elderly by a greater percentage than other age groups and which do require special moral consideration. These include:

- long term institutionalization (e.g., nursing homes)
- lack of vigorous and supportive immediate family members
- poverty
- dementia

Each of these conditions renders the sufferer especially vulnerable to abuse, including abuse in research participation.

Long term institutionalization opens several possibilities for immoral treatment. First, by being institutionalized, these persons become extremely convenient research subjects. Many subjects can be visited or treated in the same convenient location, and follow-up is very successful since such persons tend to remain readily available. This great convenience means that researchers may develop a preference for choosing such individuals far out of proportion to the population at large. Furthermore, by being institutionalized for the long term, such individuals may be seen, by themselves as well as by researchers, as a captive audience with no real choice but to accept their role as participators in research. Their moral autonomy, fragile to begin with, is threatened even further.

A lack of close and vigorous family members can render the individual vulnerable to abuse. By not having trusted family members to consult with or to question and advocate on their behalf, the individual may be too easily swayed by the persistence, insistence, and enthusiasm of the researcher.

Poverty, a condition which afflicts many elderly persons, renders the individual vulnerable by creating the feeling on the part of the individual and the researcher that participation in research is requisite in compensation for the subsidized medical care. Poor persons may even come to believe that unless they agree to participate they will not receive full and appropriate medical treatment from their physicians.

Dementia, which afflicts the elderly more than other age groups, makes research participation ethically problematic on several grounds. First, if an elderly patient of diminished competence has not been declared *legally* incompetent, medical personnel may find it convenient and easy to gain "consent" even though the patient does not understand the implications of research participation. More ethically complex, however, is the role of surrogate decision makers for enrollment (or lack of enrollment) in research. To what extent does a surrogate decision maker have the right to place an incompetent elderly person at risk in a research project? We believe that lacking evidence of the patient's willingness (expressed when competent) to participate in research that is non-therapeutic and involves risk, one ought to avoid use of incompetent participants for the most part. Respect for these persons of diminished capacity indicates that where alternate research subjects are available, effort should be made to avoid non-therapeutic interference in their lives. An obvious exception to this general rule is research that involves dementia itself, and which for that reason can only be carried out on persons suffering from dementia. In such a case, it may be ethically appropriate to involve such individuals in research that is non-therapeutic and perhaps even risky for them but which may gain information which could prove beneficial for future victims of dementia. Here, the health professional's moral duties to the public at large may outweigh the moral obligation to do no harm to the individual patient.

Melnick, et al. (1984), present guidelines for research with Alzheimer's patients in particular. It is beyond the scope of our present concern to present those guidelines in their entirety, but it is worth noting the areas of their concern. They include:

- The selection process—favoring non-institutionalized subjects over institutionalized and favoring earlier stage senile dementia of the Alzheimer's type over later stage.
- Qualification of institutional site—if institutionalized patients must be used, the site should comply with all state and federal regulations and requirements.
- Encouraged use of durable power of attorney— researchers should be encouraged to use advance directives to protect and sustain the autonomy of their subjects before the dementia progresses too far for competent decisions.
- Long term projects—researchers should be encouraged to use long-term protocols where valid consent can be obtained at early stages of dementia.
- Determination of subject's competency—researchers may wish to distinguish between a subject's legal competency and competency to consent to research participation. The law, however, is not in favor of such distinctions.
- Capacity to consent as related to risks—as the risks involved increase, researchers must be increasingly judicious in evaluating capacity to consent.
- Right to object—with the exception of beneficial therapy for an incompetent patient, safeguards must be in place to ensure the subject's right to refuse or withdraw from participation.
- Guardianship—use of legally designated guardians who should be able to effectively protect and advocate for the subject's interests.

We must not, however, let the increased vulnerability of the elderly block all research. As Cassel has argued (1987) and as recent examples illustrate, even in research projects which involve little or no risk and which might provide useful information, excessive concern about vulnerability and/or public mistrust of researchers and lack of understanding of its importance have hampered medical research. This is particularly true of research involving the health problems of the elderly. We must learn to strike a sensible balance between risk to the individual and benefit for the group.

6.3 Case Revisited

Fortunately, the experiences of Dr. Ratzan are not so frequent as to obviate conducting studies in either the nursing home or with the elderly. However, it is important that we pay heed to the obstacles he encountered. In geriatric medical research, there are four parties which must be addressed both individually and within their relationships: the institution, the patient, the family, and non-participating primary care physicians.

From the institutional perspective, there are several important points to consider in proposing a research agenda. First, the nature of nursing homes is one which emphasizes a nurturing, tranquil and home-like environment—a milieu of low technology and highly personal care (see chapter 13). Research is a relatively new phenomenon to this setting. It is also usually motivated from outside the institution, and therefore represents a potentially threatening intrusion. Second, cost efficiency is a major concern. Teaching hospitals routinely subsume an overhead surcharge from all grants which pass through their administration, even when the work is not done on the premises. "Hidden costs" to the nursing home must be carefully scrutinized and accounted for within the research budget. Third, the very nature of research is to question the way things are done. Although the motivation is generally noble, there develops an inevitable uncertainty about the quality of care currently rendered, with a division of opinion among the staff.

Dr. Ratzan had clearly gained the full support of the institution's administration; the constructs necessary for independent research were organized by the facility. His status as a member of the medical staff was more than likely a critical element in the success of this aspect of his study. In fact, the majority of research seems to come from facilities whose physicians are intimately involved in the planning and execution of the work and whose administrations are willing to invest their resources in its support. However, this is not always possible or practical. In these instances it is usually necessary to bring in fully dedicated personnel or to pay specific salary lines for institutional staff to conduct the data collection, in addition to assuring funding for incidental costs.

Patient selection, as well as obtaining consent, presented significant barriers. The fact that only 24 out of 107 patients were eligible reflects both the extent of dementia in the nursing home and the stringency of the mental status testing. We think it appropriate that Dr. Ratzan did not try to obtain proxy consents, which may have increased his abilities to find a suitable population, because the study was of marginal benefit to the patients involved. Any risk or intrusion would have to be kept in balance. However, had the benefits been more clear, the risks were not so onerous as to make proxy consents unethical. In fact, nearly any large-scale research will be dependent on the investigators' abilities to obtain consent from others. And, any institution which may wish to participate in research programs will need to develop their own, or agree to accept criteria for proxy consents for their mentally impaired patients.

Patient marketing was also not effective. If widespread volunteerism is to be gained, it is vital to gain support from among a few patient leaders when approaching a closed society such as a nursing home. Small group discussions, accompanied by representatives from the nursing staff, help to build a sense of contribution, purpose and camaraderie and allay concerns about the intrusiveness of the study. One can more easily identify those whose support warrants special attention for promoting general acceptance. Our experience is that when a few key individuals are willing to participate, others are more likely to follow; if not, the study should be reevaluated.

Support of the family is also a crucial factor. One reality of institutional life is that families most often have a sense of guilt because they are unable to provide the care themselves. This is usually manifest as protectionism; the degree of advocacy depends on the family's vociferousness. Therefore, it is equally important to win family approval to avoid sabotaging the consent of the competent patient as well as for proxy consent for those with mental impairments.

The last item of importance is the support of one's peers from the medical and nursing staff who are not directly involved in the research project. Acceptance is likely to be inversely correlated to the extent that the study questions establish approaches to care or raise concerns about issues currently not addressed. Uncertainty is not comfortable for many practitioners and change often difficult because it implies that less than optimal care is being, or has been, rendered. Also, a study comparing different regimens may be construed as defining a preferred method of treatment. This may be seen as constricting the physicians' choices or making them defensive in choosing another approach. However, their endorsement will help both patients and families decide in favor of participation. Just as patients and their families must be educated as to the benefits, the professional staff will need appropriate information and a chance to question or even join in the project.

Finally, the researchers must address the inter-relationships between these parties. The administration must maintain cordial dealings with the families of its clientele. Families of the current residents are a major means of marketing for prospective patients and other community supports, such as volunteers. However, there is a tenuous balance that families and the administration share around nurturing: protectionism versus cost containment. The intrusiveness of experimentation can easily upset this balance, especially if the rationale is felt to involve a lower cost approach to care. This comes from an anecdotal impression that many families have a healthy disregard for the profits of long-term care providers. Therefore, the safety and benefits must be clearly defined in order that the intrusion be mitigated and the balance reestablished.

Questions raised by research may also challenge relationships between participating and non-participating physicians and their patients or families. Although we strongly endorse an active research program within the institutional setting, physicians must be given a choice whenever possible as to the extent of their involvement, and that choice must be respected by the administration. The study question(s) must be framed so as to remove any stigma from those who choose not to be a part. This obviates the protectionism of the non-participating physicians, who seriously affected Dr. Ratzan's study. In a similar way, an attempt to maintain a neutral position on the part of the researchers will reduce friction that may develop between the physician, patient and family regarding their decisions.

In summary, clinical research with institutionalized patients presents more challenges than in nearly any other setting. But careful planning and broad-based education is very likely to be successful when the benefits-versus-risk ratio is clearly large and the costs to the institution are held within acceptable constraints.

6.4 Conclusion

Experience has shown that there is a balance to be struck between protecting the vulnerable patient, such as the institutionalized elderly, and promoting the wider interests of society. There have been periods and episodes in the history of medical research when research subjects were abused. By the same token, there have been, particularly in recent years, many valuable and worthwhile research projects which were never implemented because of overprotection of vulnerable research subjects. We have argued that persons can have a moral duty, albeit an imperfect (unenforceable) duty, to participate in responsibly designed, useful, and relatively harmless research. Though we should strive to continue to respect potential research subjects as individuals, we should also make an effort to educate our patients and the public about the importance and significance of continuing research.

Our knowledge in medicine is predicated on research. For us to better care for older people, we must develop the means to study their needs, and to make reasoned decisions based on scientific findings. Research has in many ways benefited those who are currently among the aged; it has also brought about problems in the care of the elderly which we would hope to address. However, we must also take special pains to protect those with mental impairments which compromise their free choice and to avoid the insidious pressures which result from dependency.

Annotated Bibliography

Cassel CK. "Informed Consent for Research in Geriatrics: History and Concepts," *Journal of the American Geriatric Society* 35:542–44 (1987).
Cassel argues that while there were indeed moral abuses of vulnerable patients in previous years, the current practices of

protecting research subjects are so stringent that much valuable and morally acceptable research is not being done.

References

Cassel CK. "Informed Consent for Research in Geriatrics: History and Concepts," *Journal of the American Geriatric Society* 35:542–44 (1987).

Melnick VL, Dubler NN, Weisbard A, and Butler RN. "Clinical Research in Senile Dementia of the Alzheimer Type," *Journal of the American Geriatrics Society* 32(7):531–36 (1984).

Ratzan RM. "The Experiment That Wasn't: A Case Report in Clinical Geriatric Research," *Gerontologist* 21:297–302 (1981).

Part II

Decision Making Concerning Levels of Intervention

CHAPTER 7

Diagnostic Intervention and Compromise

The Case of Mrs. Wilson

The office staff always looks forward to Mrs. Wilson's visits since her family owns a local confectionery with a well-deserved reputation for its chocolate candies. Mrs. Wilson brings a large box for the front desk and all those in the waiting area share in an impromptu party. She has enjoyed good health except for a troublesome forgetfulness and impairment of her arithmetic and language skills. She usually manages to cover these, though, with her remarkable gaiety. Her daughter accompanies her on visits "for companionship"—but actually to convey the facts of her status more realistically.

On her last annual examination, she was found to have occult blood in her stool. The barium enema revealed a suspicious lesion in the descending colon which could be ascribed to a diverticular stricture—but could also represent a carcinoma. The radiologic study was quite traumatic. Mrs. Wilson had suffered a catastrophic reaction with hysterical crying and shouting until she eventually fainted in the x-ray suite. Her daughter was concerned about the prospects of colonoscopy. Mrs. Wilson had only vague recollections of the barium enema, but obviously was not in favor of the proposed procedure as described to her.

Discussion

This chapter examines questions concerning diagnostic intervention, while subsequent chapters consider questions concerning treatment, nutrition, hydration, resuscitation, suicide, and euthanasia. More and more articles appear concerning advance directives, durable power of attorney, limited treatment plans for the elderly, and quality-of-life judgments. But precious few of these make much headway in understanding how the nature of the person, the goals of medicine, and the patient-provider relationship provide a moral context for such decision making. In these chapters, we seek to provide a philosophical understanding of when and why it may be morally correct to withhold or withdraw medical procedures and how these principles can be applied in actual medical practice.

There are several reasons for pursuing this kind of understanding.

First, it is probable that the medical professional has already faced cases involving the elderly where such issues have arisen. Some decision has been made, though the health care professional may be unclear about the reasons or ethical justifications (or objections) for this decision, prompting apprehension about facing such situations again in the future. Seeing why it can sometimes be ethically proper to withhold or withdraw diagnostic or treatment procedures can be both intellectually and emotionally helpful for the professional.

Second, even with competent patients, the health care professional must be prepared to offer such advice and be able to explain the beliefs and/or reasoning behind such advice. We have repeatedly stressed the ethical importance of seeking and respecting the wishes of the competent patient, but the patient cannot be expected to make a reasonable choice in a vacuum. The health care professional must be prepared to offer the patient ethical wisdom as well as physiological knowledge.

Third, this understanding can aid the health care professional in making recommendations concerning the care of incompetent patients. To foist the decision making completely onto the family or other guardian is to abandon the patient and place an undue burden upon the family or guardian. The health care professional must be prepared to offer intelligent, ethically sensitive, and well thought out advice.

Fourth, understanding the ethical rationale behind the advance directives or limited treatment plans which patients might choose to accept prevents the professional from being alienated from the patient and makes it easier for the professional truly to care for the patient as a suffering person.

Fifth and finally, the health care professional must have an understanding and appreciation of the issues in assisting the institutions in which they work to develop guidelines, policies, and procedures for patient caring within their own legal and financial constraints.

7.1 Limited Intervention and the Goals of Medicine

We must begin by accepting a richer conception of the goals of medicine. The practice of medicine should be not only to cure disease and prolong life, but also to relieve suffering and provide support. An overly narrow conception of the art of medicine requires aggressive intervention in cases where a more reflective and humane notion of medicine would recommend a much different course of action.

One of the things which has fostered this belief in the public at large is that physicians themselves have come to think this way. Remarkable advancements in medical science have enlarged the capacity of medicine to cure; the medical technology which makes such intervention possible occupies a larger and larger portion of medical education. Hence, the character of medical education has come to strongly encourage interventionist *action* on the part of the physician. The medical student or resident is taught how to *do* something. Rarely if ever are we taught restraint, or how to do *nothing* without abandoning our patients.

Furthermore, when we are unable to provide the hoped-for cure, we may feel as though we, as medical professionals, have somehow failed our patient.

Unfortunately, this obsession with curing is not morally benign. It fails to see the variety of ways in which medicine may appropriately serve the interests of the person. Eric J. Cassell (1982), for example, has eloquently argued that in addition to the goals of the curing of disease, medicine has the equally important goal of the relief of suffering, broadly understanding the forms that suffering may take. Suffering may arise from purely physical pain. It may also be caused by the loss of loved ones; by the loss of personal mobility; by the loss of special capacities (e.g., a pianist who has become hopelessly crippled by severe arthritis, or the elderly scholar who has lost the ability to see clearly enough to read); or by the loss of hope.

If we focus exclusively upon the curing of disease and ignore the wider dimensions of patient suffering, it is quite possible that we may end up causing more suffering in our patients than we relieve. This is particularly true of our elderly patients, for the elderly are naturally prone to chronic, debilitating and irreversible conditions. The elderly are more likely to suffer from a distressing decrease in important capabilities from diseases which restrict their lifestyle and for which there are no cures. They are most likely to have suffered the irreversible loss through death of close friends and loved ones.

Here we may see how quality-of-life judgments—judgments which many health care professionals ostensibly refuse to make—are an integral aspect of ethically sensitive medical practice. Making use of quality-of-life considerations is not, as many health care professionals believe, a matter of passing judgment upon the *value* of certain persons. Instead, it is a means for allowing us to see beyond a diagnose-and-cure orientation toward the caring for the person as a whole. It allows us to ask whether or not by treating a specific condition we are actually benefiting the person.

What holds true for treatment decisions in general also holds true for diagnostic procedures. Yet there has been little discussion in the literature concerning the ethics of refraining from diagnostic interventions. Nevertheless, this is an ethical issue which must be addressed because diagnostic interventions are not themselves completely benign. Invasive procedures can inflict significant physical suffering upon a patient. Even when not technically invasive, diagnostic procedures can disrupt a patient's life, causing inconvenience and aggravation. And even in the case of non-invasive and minimally disruptive diagnostic procedures, there is a financial cost to be considered. Since diagnostic procedures can cause suffering, just as treatment procedures, whether to apply a certain procedure is an ethically laden choice. A starting point is to delineate the reasons for considering a diagnostic test.

7.2 The Pros and Cons of Diagnostic Intervention

Before making an informed ethical judgment on why a certain diagnostic procedure should or should not be performed, it is necessary to understand what the ethical values are and how the diagnostic intervention fits into those values. Usually, what is faced is a conflict between the possible benefit to the patient of the diagnostic procedure and the possible risk or suffering which the intervention might entail. Patient welfare is what is at question. As health care professionals we know that in most cases something positive may be gained from an accurate diagnosis, something that might influence a treatment plan. It is cases where the diagnostic procedure will be inconvenient or cause suffering but may also open up the possibility for beneficial treatment that the health care professional faces ethically difficult choices. Let us begin by considering the possible benefits to be had by diagnostic intervention.

Benefits of diagnostic intervention: One reason for performing a diagnostic procedure is to define a disease process which will significantly affect quantity or quality of life, for which cure and/or palliation is available, and is wanted. In the same vein, one may wish to perform a diagnostic procedure to monitor a disease process currently under treatment for the same reasons noted above.

Second, one may want to identify a disease process for clarification of its clinical course and prognosis. The information may prove useful in allowing the physician to anticipate developments in the patient's condition and to prepare the patient for future developments.

Third, one may choose to perform a diagnostic procedure for the simple reason that the patient wants to know—an understandable desire. Insofar as is legitimately possible, the health care provider has a moral obligation to assist the patient in discovering this information.

Fourth, the family may have a need to know. This is particularly true where the patient is being cared for in the home and the family will have to prepare itself (psychologically, financially, logistically, etc.) for the kind of care demands that will arise naturally over the course of a diagnosed disease process. This is also true where there is the potential for communicable or inheritable disease.

Fifth, society may have a right to know. Good health statistics are an important element of promoting public health and hygiene. The legitimate interests of society at large may require a diagnostic intervention even in circumstances where the patient will not benefit from the identification of the disease and its stage of progress.

Sixth, diagnostic intervention may be performed for the sake of educational purposes, for example, for the training of medical students and student nurses.

Harms of diagnostic intervention: The harms associated with diagnostic intervention are varied. One level is financial restraint. Diagnostic interventions can be expensive, and the patient may consider the expense to him or herself too heavy a price to pay. A second level of harm is the suffering associated with inconvenience, embarrassment, and discomfort. This suffering may range from minimal (e.g., the taking of blood samples) to quite severe (e.g., endoscopy, tissue biopsy or surgical exploration). A third level of harm is the risk involved with interventions (e.g., adverse reactions). In an effort to remind the health care professional that patient suffering *is* associated with most diagnostic interventions, we suggest the following categorization which provides a rough ranking according to degrees of harm.

> 1) Readily accessible with no significant risks: These procedures can be performed with minimal inconvenience to the patient and cause minimal suffering (physical or emotional).
> 2) Disruptive or minimally invasive or involving some risk: These procedures may require some disruption of the patient's life (e.g., fasting, travel, disrobing in public) and may be minimally invasive (e.g., IV enhancement dyes, sigmoidoscopy, gastroscopy, or biopsies).
> 3) Invasive or involving substantial risk: These procedures require the surgical opening of the body or deep penetration of bodily orifices (e.g., laparotomy, colonoscopy, pelvic evaluation under anesthesia).

Examples of readily accessible procedures are taking vital signs, venepuncture, and urinalysis. These can be performed with virtually no patient suffering.

Disruptive or minimally invasive procedures could include such procedures as the taking of x-rays, CTscans, sonograms, sigmoidoscopy or skin biopsies. These procedures require no invasive insertions into the body, but do require the patient to come to a specific and often inconvenient location for the procedure. It also often requires the embarrassment of removing clothes and physical discomforts.

Finally, invasive diagnostic procedures include (but are by no means limited to) such interventions as surgical biopsy, surgical explorations, and spinal punctures.

The crucial question, of course, is, *considering the suffering which a diagnostic intervention will probably cause, would we or would we not be doing the patient a "favor" by doing it?* Will the information gained from the diagnostic procedure provide us with the means to relieve the patient's suffering to such an extent that the patient is more than compensated for the suffering caused by the diagnostic intervention?

There can be no simple answers as each case will involve the care of a unique individual. The possible value of a diagnostic procedure may vary from the perspective of the physicians and the patient. In addition, the value to the patient must be balanced with the suffering of the individual in his or her own terms. This would include such straightforward factors as the patient's overall physical condition (e.g., there might be serious additional health problems which make the diagnosis of a concomitant problem beside the point) and less obvious factors, such as the patient's psychosocial outlook and values.

In guiding decision making for incompetent patients or in offering advice to competent patients, we are primarily concerned with overall patient welfare. Thus, it is morally proper to recognize a balance between the suffering caused by intervention and the probable benefits gained. When suffering is greater than anticipated benefits, the diagnostic intervention should be foregone. (See the discussion related to this in chapter 2.) We believe that the health care professional should hold a moderate view of where this dividing line between intervention and non-intervention should be drawn, except in those cases where the health care professional agrees otherwise with a competent patient or is directed by previously expressed wishes. We should be sensitive to the suffering of our patients, in the many forms that it might take. And we should recognize that the minimization of that suffering is one important goal of the practice of medicine.

7.3 Reaching a Decision Concerning Diagnostic Intervention

We suggest three stages in reaching decisions concerning whether or not to intervene with diagnostic procedures. First, the issue must be raised. Second, the health care team, and if necessary the institutional administration, should discuss the matter. And third, the results of the team's discussion should be presented to the patient, family, or guardian with the aim of reaching a coherent consensus.

Raising the issue: One can imagine four typical ways that the issue of whether or not to proceed with a diagnostic procedure might arise. First the physician or any other team member may be uncomfortable with the thought of proceeding with what appears to be the standard diagnostic procedure. Second, the patient himself may be disinclined to proceed. Third, the family may express opposition to the contemplated procedure. Fourth, the institutional administration may oppose the procedure.

It is not necessary that the person who has doubts about the wisdom or appropriateness of the procedure have a clearly formulated and articulated understanding at this stage of the process of why he or she is not happy with the contemplated intervention. "Gut instincts" should not be final arbiters of moral matters, but they do merit serious attention. They can be like fire alarms—sometimes they can be mistaken, but sometimes they can detect a problem before we are aware of it. Such qualms or doubts deserve further investigation.

Clarifying and assessing the issue: Once doubts have been raised about the moral appropriateness of a diagnostic intervention, the question should be brought before the health care team. The team needs to review several things:

- What are the risks, physiological and psychological, of the diagnostic intervention?
- What therapeutic alternatives might become appropriate because of a confirmed diagnosis?
- What are the therapeutic alternatives without the knowledge to be gained from the diagnostic intervention?
- What legal issues might be involved, both with respect to the health care team and the health care institution?
- What are the patient's (or the family's) values relating

to the various alternatives? (The answer to this question should be based upon information gained *from* the patient or family, not from "hunches" or presumptions.)

- What are the values of the physician and the team that relate to this matter? Are they different from, or congruent with, the patient's values?
- Who is morally and legally responsible for the final decision? (Is the patient competent? Is there a legally appointed guardian?)
- Are the resources available (in physical and monetary terms) for doing the diagnostic procedure and offering treatment?

Presenting the Issues: After discussing the issues noted above, the health care team should seek to formulate a recommendation to present to the patient. This recommendation should be designed to assist the patient (where competent) in making an informed choice. It should not be composed with the idea of determining the patient's choice by suggesting only one option (while ignoring other plausible options). Informed consent requires patient understanding, hence the recommendation of the health care team should note the alternatives and their implications. Furthermore, these recommendations should note any team dissent from the majority and its reasoning.

The presentation to the patient (guardian or family) should include information on the following:

- Benefits: What are the possible or probable benefits to be gained from the diagnostic intervention? What knowledge is to be gained? What therapeutic options become available? Will the knowledge make a reasonably accurate prognosis possible?
- Risks and suffering: What are the risks or harms of the intervention? What adverse consequences might develop? What pain and discomfort will result from the invasiveness of the procedure? What is the time frame of potential suffering?
- Location: What will be the setting for the intervention? Can inconvenience be minimized by doing the procedure in the home? Can the procedure be done in the physician's office? Or must it be done in the hospital or some other special setting?
- Inconveniences: If the test is not to be done where the patient currently is, what sort of transportation is available or can be arranged?

- Financial considerations: What costs are involved? Particularly, what is the share of costs which will be borne by the patient?

Reaching a Decision: Once the presentation is made to the patient (or the morally responsible party if the patient is incompetent), then consensual agreement between the patient and the health care professionals should be sought. Great effort should be made to resolve any differences of opinion at this level. If that is not possible, the next appropriate step would be to seek counsel from the institutional ethics committee. Failing resolution here, the health care team may withdraw from the case if doing so would not constitute abandonment. Judicial intervention may be sought as a last resort, especially if the welfare of an incompetent patient hangs in the balance.

7.4 Case Revisited

The physician sensed hesitance on the part of the daughter and the patient in pursuing the colonoscopy as planned and realized that, in order to proceed, a patient/family conference would need to be held to more clearly raise the issues involved in the decision. The gastroenterologist was called and the problems outlined. The consultation revealed that although the procedure was recommended in the complete evaluation of occult bleeding, the likelihood of uncovering a significantly new finding was small. In fact, the possibility of perforating the bowel in an uncooperative patient probably obviated the benefits; it would be difficult to justify general anesthesia for what is intrinsically a screening procedure. The more immediate risks of an impending obstruction were, in fact, excluded by the barium enema.

The physician also considered the consequences of a suspicious finding and recognized that although the gastroenterologist would have accepted her permission for colonoscopy, she was not of sufficient mental capability to sign an informed consent for exploratory surgery. The requirement for guardianship would also need to become a part of the diagnostic plan.

The physician then presented the alternatives to the patient and her daughter. Neither were interested in pursuing the colonoscopy and the physician accepted their decision, although with some reservation. The possibilities of a significant finding, though remote, remained troublesome. The issues of advance directives were then raised. Mrs. Wilson was quite clear that she felt she had lived a good life and enjoyed herself, but was concerned about becoming a burden to her children. All agreed that a Living Will was an appropriate consideration and they were given a form to take home and discuss with the rest of the family. The physician made clear to both Mrs. Wilson and her daughter that the decision to refuse intervention did not mean that their relationship was over. He and the rest of the health care team would continue to care for her.

7.5 Conclusion

There has been a tendency in medical education to emphasize interventions by the health care professional. Certain clinical observations or suspicions automatically dictate a pattern of diagnostic tests. The health care profession is gradually realizing, though, that such diagnostic interventions are not necessarily good medical practice. In particular cases, these interventions may not produce any useful knowledge. Moreover, in some cases they may cause undue pain and suffering, or be contrary to the values of either the patient or the physician.

It is too simplistic to conclude that whenever pain and suffering are foreseeable consequences of diagnostic intervention, the intervention should be foregone. The information gained from diagnostic intervention can be of substantial benefit to either the patient or to society, even when it is invasive and directly causes suffering. The aim must be to recognize a balancing point beyond which the suffering and risk inherent in the intervention outweigh the expected benefits. The decision process concerning diagnostic intervention must not only bring to light the benefits and harms of a proposed procedure for a particular patient. The decision must be reached in such a way that the autonomy of the patient is respected and the professional and ethical integrity of each member of the health care team is preserved.

Annotated Bibliography

President's Commission for the Study of Ethical Problems in Medicine and Biomedical and Behavioral Research, *Making*

Health Care Decisions, US Government Printing Office, 1982.

—*Deciding to Forego Life-Sustaining Treatment*, US Government Printing Office, 1983.

These are two of the many well-known volumes issued by the President's Commission. Both are very important texts which should be a part of any physician's or health care institution's library.

References

Braithwaite S, and Thomasma DC. "New Guidelines on Foregoing Life-Sustaining Treatment in Incompetent Patients: An Anti-Cruelty Policy." *Annals of Internal Medicine* 104:711–15 (1986).

Cassell EJ. "The Nature of Suffering and the Goals of Medicine." *New England Journal of Medicine* 306(11): 639–45 (1982).

CHAPTER 8

Levels of Treatment

The Case of Mr. Pimm

"Mr. Pimm was followed for lung cancer at home by the hospice team until he became too disabled from radiation treatments to care for himself. At the recommendation of the nurse, he elected admission to the inpatient hospice program at our long-term care facility for an intended short stay. During the initial patient care conference, Mr. Pimm expressed his wish to discontinue his radiation treatments and "beat this on my own." The radiation oncologist was consulted and agreed that whatever benefit could be offered had probably been achieved, and that Mr. Pimm was not under any specific research protocols. This accomplished, he settled in and began to regain his appetite and strength.

"Plans were being made for Mr. Pimm to return home when he awoke one morning with back pain. X-rays and a bone scan suggested widespread bony metastases and a pathologic fracture of a mid-thoracic vertebra. The radiation oncologist felt that further treatments would not be helpful since maximal dosage had already been given to the area. Palliative medical therapy was therefore instituted.

"At the second patient care conference, the options for treatment of potential illness were discussed. The issues of intensive care were easily dispensed with since Mr. Pimm emphatically stated his wish not to be placed on a ventilator. He stated that he had no preference to be alert up to the time of death but wished that he be allowed to die quietly. We negotiated a do-not-hospitalize agreement by assuring him that intravenous medications, oxygen and respiratory therapy were available at the hospice— identical to those available on the ward of the acute care hospital. He was not in favor of nasogastric intubation should he be unable to eat, having seen several patients fed this way. Mr. Pimm also allowed that the team should make decisions for him if for some reason he became unable.

"The medical regimen was effective for several months except for an episode of partial intestinal obstruction attributed to the narcotics. This was managed with nasogastric suction, IV hydration and decreased dosages of opiates. When it passed, the tube and IV were removed and adjuvant therapy prescribed for added pain control. Unfortunately, he never fully recovered and his decline became more noticeable.

"Approximately one week later, Mr. Pimm suffered a marked change in status, with fever, upper respiratory congestion, and confusion. Chest x-ray confirmed the clinical diagnosis of a post-obstructive pneumonia. According to his wishes, IV hydration was reinstituted, and antibiotics and oxygen administered; he was too confused and agitated for nebulizer treatments. After the fifth day, the nurse reported that she could no longer gain intravenous access. The physician was called and one dose of intramuscular antibiotics was ordered and a team conference scheduled. It was agreed that treatment of the pneumonia was not succeeding as hoped and that therapy be withdrawn. No further IVs or antibiotics were given; pain medications by injection, though made available, were never needed. Mr. Pimm died the following morning."

Discussion

In caring for the elderly, health care professionals often face the question of whether or not a certain form of treatment is appropriate for a particular patient, even when there is a firm diagnosis and a corresponding standard treatment regimen. Nor is it only health care professionals who sometimes have doubts about these matters; often patients themselves, or their families or guardians, will wonder about and ask the same sort of question. We suggested in the preceding chapter that under certain circumstances health care professionals may refrain from using some diagnostic procedures. In this chapter we suggest that this also holds true for treatment.

Discussion of limited treatment as a subject separate from limited use of diagnostic intervention is justified for several reasons. First, there is a symbolic distinction. Treatment, whether for good reasons or not, is more closely associated with caring than diagnostic intervention. Second, the motives are importantly different. Diagnostic intervention is motivated by a desire to acquire knowledge; treatment is motivated by a desire to change a patient's condition. Third, unlike seeking a firm diagnosis, treatment (especially in the care of the elderly) tends to be a long-term proposition. Thus, the suffering as a result of the intervention may well be over a prolonged period of time. Fourth, more so than with diagnostic procedures, there is a danger of a "snowball" effect with therapeutic intervention escalating far beyond initial expectations as the illness continues its natural course. For these reasons, decisions on whether or not to treat deserve special consideration.

8.1 What Is Limited Treatment?

The health care professional will already be familiar with some rudimentary forms of limited treatment, such as orders not to resuscitate (DNR). Succeeding chapters will examine more specifically DNR orders and decisions not to artificially feed and hydrate. This chapter will deal with limited treatment in more general terms.

There is a great deal of confusion and misunderstanding concerning limited treatment orders. To develop a working definition of limited treatment, one must first understand what limited treatment is not.

1) *Limited treatment does not mean "no treatment."* The decision not to pursue a standard treatment regimen for one illness should have no bearing on other patient problems. Too frequently

we have seen or heard reports of medical staff not giving a patient any treatment only because it had been decided to withhold one specific form of treatment (such as CPR). This is a gross misunderstanding of limited treatment, and leads to highly unethical medical practice. Limited treatment usually does not imply refraining from treatment of reversible conditions or inattention to comfort measures. Nor does it mean ineligibility for physical therapy or corrective surgery.

2) *Limited treatment usually does not aim to encourage or hasten death.* It is true that limited treatment may occasionally result in death sooner than full treatment, but represents a balance between the quality and quantity of life. Almost all limited treatment plans seek to maintain life, but *only under acceptable conditions.* Limited treatment should not be understood as euthanasia or intentionally hastening death but as treatment plans designed to help patients *live on their own terms.*

3) *Limited treatment does not mean ceasing to care.* A decision to limit treatment should be understood as a decision to withhold or withdraw *certain kinds* of medical intervention, not as an abandonment. Instead, it is a decision that palliation, emotional support, and counseling shall predominate over efforts to cure.

A limited treatment plan is motivated by a conscious decision to target treatment toward certain goals chosen by the patient (or patient surrogate) and to *restrict* treatment to those forms which are consistent with these specified goals. It is an overt statement of decision processes which are, in fact, made in everyday clinical practice. What those kinds of interventions are to be, as well as the purpose behind the restrictions, must be clearly indicated in the limited treatment plan. To fail to be clear concerning the terms of limited treatment invites misunderstanding and misinterpretation on the part of the patient, family, and members of the health care team.

8.2 Why Have Limited Treatment?

There are three basic reasons for choosing to limit the level of treatment intervention:

1) The futility of treatment in the context of the patient's overall condition
2) Quality-of-life considerations (as determined by the

competent patient, or by appropriate others for the incompetent patient)
3) High costs or scarce resources.

Let us consider each of these in turn.

1) Futility of treatment

The health care professional clearly has no obligation (ethical or professional) to administer futile treatment. This is a position that has been advocated by the President's Commission (1983) and endorsed by the AMA. If a particular kind of treatment will not promote the health and well-being of the patient, the health care professional has no moral obligation to provide such treatment. In fact, it is more easily understood as *contrary* to medical ethics to administer useless or futile treatment. Doing so is not only a waste of health care resources, which may adversely affect others who could benefit more, but it may also foster mistaken hope in the patient or the patient's family.

2) Quality-of-life considerations

Inevitably, quality-of-life considerations play a role whenever decisions are made to withhold or withdraw certain therapies. Nonetheless, many health care professionals are disturbed by the thought of allowing quality-of-life considerations to play a role in decisions concerning treatment or non-treatment. (See, for example, Koop CE, 1978.) This disposition to avoid or condemn the use of quality-of-life considerations arises from two arguments.

First, some argue that there is no objective scale of quality-of-life. Empirical evidence indicates that health care professionals themselves have widely differing views on what constitutes an appropriate quality-of-life consideration (Pearlman RA and Jonsen A, 1985). They take this to indicate that we cannot rise above our subjective biases to make objective and impartial quality-of-life judgments. Thus, they conclude, health care professionals should refrain from making quality-of-life judgments and should refuse to let such judgments play a role in decisions about treatment or non-treatment. Second, some argue that the very sanctity of life demands that we must do whatever possible to *preserve* life and not hasten death by withholding or withdrawing treatment.

Let us discuss these objections in turn. Quality of life is a very subjective measure because it is based upon the experiences of individual subjects. What is acceptable to one person may seem unacceptable to another. What is important to one person may be trivial to another. What causes unbearable suffering in one may cause only mild inconvenience to another (Cassell EJ, 1982). Nevertheless, the inherent subjectivity of quality-of-life considerations should not be regarded as a reason for forbidding quality-of-life judgments.

Given that quality of life is a subjective matter, it is the patient who is best suited to judge what he or she finds personally acceptable or unacceptable. Yet this decision is not solely a matter of patient wishes. Any such decision requires some medical expertise to know whether such suffering can be ameliorated by therapy or whether a proposed treatment would merely prolong suffering. Decisions to limit treatment determine how the health care team will care for the patient. The nature of the treatment choices of the patient may conflict with the moral commitments of the health care team. There ought, therefore, to be a consensus between the competent patient and the health care providers. If consensus cannot be reached, the patient or providers may choose to seek care elsewhere (or by another practitioner), providing that doing so would not constitute abandonment.

The use of quality-of-life considerations in the care of incompetent individuals (who have left no advance directives prior to incompetency) is complicated by the subjectivity of these considerations. Cases where there is no reliable evidence of what a patient would want are ethically the most troublesome. Most frequently this involves persons who have never discussed these issues or who have been distant from their family members for some time or who do not have family members. In the former, family members are no longer reliable guides to how the patient would prefer to be treated now. In the latter, there may be no one known to the medical staff who ever knew the patient before he or she became mentally incompetent.

In these cases some ethicists, such as Ramsey, have argued that quality-of-life considerations should not be allowed to play any real role, for to allow anyone other than patients themselves to make that decision is morally mistaken.

> Both covenant fidelity to the life and interests of another as well as the stringency of fiduciary obligations of familial or medical or legal guardianship require that a medical indications policy alone be applied when another, voiceless, human life is at stake. (1978, 161)

The danger, in Ramsey's mind, is that a proxy might find an incompetent patient's life not worth living, whereas the patient, *if he were able to express his feelings,* would argue that he is sufficiently happy with his condition to wish to continue to live, even if to do so requires medical intervention

While we must not deny that a younger, fully competent designated proxy may in some instances have a higher standard of what constitutes a minimally acceptable quality of life than that which an older patient might be willing to accept, we should also hesitate to deny to the incompetent patient access to that course of action (or inaction) which could minimize suffering and maximize human dignity. We must seek some standard for making quality-of-life decisions for withholding treatment in such cases which recognizes and accounts for the particulars of the elderly patient involved. One suggestion which we have already had occasion to endorse is that of Thomasma (1986). He argues that treatment decisions for the elderly incompetent, for whom we have no known expression of desire from when they were competent, should be based upon the kinds of choices recommended by competent elderly patients in similar circumstances. We think this argument has a great deal of merit. Perhaps more practical is the use of institutional ethics committees to offer advice from the perspectives of a variety of persons who have been trained in ethical decision making. Another option, and one which may currently be legally required in several states, is judicial review.

Finally, it should be noted that non-treatment because of quality-of-life considerations need not be restricted to patients suffering from terminal diseases, nor need death be imminent. The AMA's Council on Ethical and Judicial Affairs (1986) has endorsed the view that competent patients may themselves decide if the proposed treatment or the foreseeable results of the treatment are unacceptable. It also states that treatment may properly be withheld from irreversibly comatose patients by consensual agreement between all responsible parties involved when it is felt that no real human benefit can be gained. This is allowable even when the patient does not suffer from a terminal condition which makes death imminent. Thus:

> Even if death is not imminent but a patient's coma is beyond doubt irreversible and there are adequate safeguards to confirm the accuracy of the diagnosis and with the concurrence of those who have responsibility

for the care of the patient, it is not unethical to discontinue all means of life prolonging medical treatment. (AMA, 1986)

The most difficult decisions in clinical practice are those involving non-terminal but incompetent patients who suffer from severe and irreversible dementia. As Hilfiker notes (1983), there are many patients who, while not comatose, suffer from severe and irreversible cognitive debility. It is arguable whether or not treating such patients with any other purpose than relieving suffering and maintaining comfort is ethically proper. The loss of human dignity which such patients face, combined with the inability to interact in a cognitive fashion with other persons, may well constitute an overall balance of suffering or undesirable indignity. Maintaining the biological lives of these patients through extraordinary interventions is difficult to justify as beneficence.

For these sorts of reasons, Braithwaite and Thomasma (1986) argue that an "anti-cruelty policy" can justify the withholding or withdrawing of treatment, even life-sustaining treatment.* They argue that such considerations are appropriate when a patient has a "hopeless injury," by which they mean:

> . . . a condition in which there is no potential for growth or repair; no observable pleasure or happiness in living aside from immediate and transitory physical satisfaction; and a total absence of one or more of the following attributes of quality of life: cognition or recognition, motor activity, memory or awareness of time, consciousness, and language or other intelligent means of communicating thoughts or wishes.

To persist in treating an incompetent patient under these circumstances is only to perpetuate the injury and therefore constitutes a form of cruelty. It directly violates the moral maxim that we should "above all, do no harm." This view is also reflected in the AMA's statement that:

---

*Braithwaite and Thomasma put forward their argument as a guideline for determining treatment for incompetent patients, but by natural extension should surely sanction such treatment by health care professionals when requested by competent patients.

In deciding what is in the best interests of the patient who is incompetent to act in his own behalf, the physician should determine what the possibility is for extending life *under humane and comfortable conditions* and what are the prior expressed wishes of the patient and attitudes of the family or those who have responsibility for the custody of the patient. (AMA, 1986)

3) Costs

Considerations of costs also have an ethically legitimate role to play in decisions to limit treatment. There is a price to pay for health care services, a price which must be borne by either society or the individual.

Governmental policies should reflect the interests and concerns of all its citizens. The cost of health care availability has come to prominence through the cost-restricting mechanisms of DRGs. A logical corollary must be the consideration of distributive justice in the allocation of those resources. It is becoming of greater moral concern as to when to properly limit the kinds of treatment and/or the duration of treatment available to certain patients. There are three ways in which consideration of scarcity of resources and costs can be relevant decision-making factors: (1) at the level of social policy, (2) by the physician, and (3) by the patient.

(1) The vast increase in the numbers of the elderly, who as a group suffer from illness more than other groups, raises questions of what is a morally just allocation of health care resources. As a citizen, the health care professional should take a role in helping to formulate public policy. As a practicing professional, the existing policies must be accepted. Our aim in this study is to focus upon clinical issues. Therefore, we shall refrain from the public policy debate. (For a provocative discussion of allocation issues relating to health care for the elderly, see Daniel Callahan's *Setting Limits*, 1987.)

(2) Traditional American conceptions of the physician-patient relationship hold that the physician should always hold paramount the interest of his or her patient as an individual. The physician is to act as the patient's advocate. To allow the physician to withhold treatment from an individual patient because of finan-

cial costs that will be borne by others is to compromise the physician-patient relationship. It creates a conflict of interest and undermines the patient's trust. We suspect that this conception of the physician-patient relationship is based more on mythology than fact. But whether or not this was the case in the past, it is an issue that must be faced now and in the coming years.

It is unrealistic to believe that governmental policy, representing broad social concerns, can foresee or take into account all the possible permutations or complexities of the clinical setting. The health care professional, particularly the physician, must make an effort to understand not only the letter of the law, but its spirit.

This tension is represented in the *Ethics Manual* of the American College of Physicians (1984). At one point in the *Manual* (p. 19), one finds that the physician has a special obligation "To be aware of limitations of health service resources, such as material and personnel, and to participate with others in exercising restraint in the expenditure of these resources." The physician is also "To be aware of the costs of care and to provide care in the most efficient manner." On the other hand, the *Manual* also states (p. 31) that, "In the final analysis, no external factors should interfere with the dedication of the physician to provide optimal care for his patient." It is easy to imagine clinical circumstances where one cannot have it both ways.

Many physicians will find it difficult to withhold treatment for reasons of costs or relative scarcity of equipment. They may find it abhorrent. But the consequences of getting everything possible for an individual patient will mean that less governmental money and equipment will be available for other patients who might receive much more benefit from those resources. Real and significant harm can be done to other persons.

We have focused our attention in this study upon ethical decision making in the clinical context. We have not broached the topic of limiting treatment for the elderly in terms of social policy, that is, the *rationing* of health care services. That issue has, however, become a matter of public debate. In his recent book, *Setting Limits: Medical Goals in an Aging Society* (1987), Callahan points out that as a consequence of improved public health and hygiene, as well as advances in medical technology, the size of the elderly population has increased dramatically, both in absolute numbers and as a percentage of the population. This increase means that the elderly will present a greatly increased demand for health care services in coming years. Callahan's concern is that this potentially limitless demand for health care for the elderly could vastly diminish the amount of public resources that can be devoted to care for other segments of the population, such as pre-natal care. His conclusion is that insofar as health care is a matter of social policy and social expenditure it should be allocated in such a way as to benefit society as a whole. This, he argues, can best be done by recognizing that the future of our society depends upon the nurture of those who are young now, not upon the aged who have already had a full life. Highly technological, highly ex-pensive health care should be reserved for the young and middle aged. The elderly should be allotted only palliative care.

While we share Callahan's view that our society has paid at-tention to the extending of life without carefully considering the quality of that life, we find some of his most central conclusions disturbing. For one thing, it is our experience that chronological age alone is not a good indicator of where a particular elderly per-son stands with respect to quality of life or social contribution. To choose a chronological age, as Callahan would have us do, would inevitably exclude many vibrant, happy, and socially engaged per-sons from therapeutic treatment. By the same token, it apparently would also include many elderly persons who would not benefit much from medical intervention. Furthermore, despite Callahan's persistent attempts to assert the contrary, such a health care policy would naturally be interpreted by many people as saying that the elderly are no longer valuable as persons.

Callahan is right that this is a crucial matter of public policy, with the health and well-being of society as a whole at stake. It is an issue of great social importance which must be debated in a ra-tional and constructive manner, and a public consensus must be reached.

Though the clinician morally ought to keep in mind the health care needs of others when making decisions involving the use of expensive or scarce resources, his decision should be guided by agreed-upon social policy, not upon social policy that might in the future be agreed upon.

(3) As the government has become less willing and less able to pay all costs, more and more of the financial burden is being shifted back to the individual patient. The physician must recog-nize that respect for patient autonomy includes respecting the right and responsibility of the patient to make decisions about

how his or her wealth will be spent. To decide presumptively what the patient will (or will not) pay for would be to act paternalistically under morally inappropriate circumstances.

The patient's decision to refuse treatment because of costs can be a difficult decision for the health care professional (a person by profession committed to health care service delivery) to accept. Nevertheless, it is not necessarily irrational or immoral for elderly patients to decide that there are other things they would prefer to do with their financial resources than to pay for a treatment intervention which might prolong life for only a short time or under unhappy conditions. They may think that their money would be better spent on their grandchildren's education or by donating it to a particular charity to which they have long been committed.

Prolonged life, even if one of reasonable health, is not the only goal of most persons, including young persons. The health care professional must accept that health is only one value or goal among many.

8.3 The Limited Treatment Plan

The ideal mechanism for limiting treatment is the limited treatment plan. This is a plan developed through discussion and eventual consensus involving both the patient (when competent, otherwise family or guardian) and the health care team. Since such a plan is forward looking, it should also be noted that events may not materialize as anticipated. The patient may change his or her mind. The treatment plan is subject to change.

Steven H. Miles (1987) argues that a clearly thought out limited treatment plan can be helpful for several different reasons:

> 1) It should develop a "coherent" plan. Thus, rather than being chaotic, ad hoc, and irrational, the properly developed limited treatment plan will make clear the rationale behind the limitation of treatment. It will become clear why specific types of intervention are to be included or excluded and why.
> 2) It can allow the patient to see that the health care team still cares for the patient even though they may not apply all available intervention. The patient is not being abandoned.
> 3 A coherent plan assists all members of the health care

team to understand what kinds of treatment are (and
are not) to be used.
4) Such a plan provides evidence to patients, family, etc.
that the patient is receiving attention and care.

8.4 Developing a Limited Treatment Plan

Limited treatment plans reflect human values. They are rarely, if
ever, simple medical decisions. A limited treatment plan involves
not only the patient being treated, but also the health care team
providing the treatment. Ideally, the development of a limited
treatment plan should be a cooperative effort between the patient
and the health care team and should be acceptable to the institution.

The Patient: One aim behind the limited treatment plan is the
furtherance of patient autonomy. This purpose implies that the
health care professional should work in ways that will promote
patient autonomy in the formulation of the treatment plan. First, if
the patient is to make effective choices, then he or she must have
relevant information. But such information is not ordinarily available to the patient without assistance. It is the health care professional's obligation, as a *skilled professional with a special body of
expertise*, to share with the patient a fair, accurate representation
of the medical facts, the various treatment options, and the probable outcomes of the various options.

Second, the health care professional, particularly the physician, must not coerce the patient into a particular decision. We all
know that by a selective (though not necessarily false) presentation of the facts, including threatening or disparaging tones of
voice, we can often manipulate patients' decisions. By using such
tactics one can go through the motions of informed consent without reaching the reality of informed consent. Genuine efforts to
obtain informed consent require freely expressing one's own
views, but doing so in a non-coercive manner.

Third, it is usually not sufficient to present the patient with
the facts and await a reasoned decision. Many patients will find it
difficult to articulate their own values and to incorporate those
values into a treatment plan. The health care professional should
make every effort to help the patient express his or her values and
to work with the patient to create a treatment plan which promotes those values as much as possible.

The Team: As noted above, the health care team is involved in the limited treatment plan since it is they who will provide patient care within the restrictions of the plan. For two reasons, therefore, team members should be familiar with the treatment plan and, to some extent, should participate in formulating the plan.

First, there is the possibility that the professional mission of particular members of the team will be at odds with the patient's own values. We may be willing to give patients wide latitude in treatment choices, but we may also at some point insist upon "drawing a line." Since it would be morally wrong to demand of team members that they seriously compromise their own ethical integrity, they must be consulted as the plan develops.

Second, if the team is to consistently provide care within the framework of a specific limited treatment plan, it is necessary that they know both the plan as written and the rationale behind the written formulation.

The Institution: Health care professionals must respect the moral views of the institutions within which they practice. In formulating a limited treatment plan with a patient, they must keep in mind moral boundaries set by the institution.

We recommend that team meetings be held when possible with the patient, physician, nurse and social worker at crucial points in the treatment process. Additional team members should also be encouraged to attend as appropriate. The format of the meeting ought to be determined beforehand by the professional staff, with discussion of the options and formulation of a recommended care plan. It is advisable to record the major issues of the discussion so that this can be used as an agenda for the meeting with the patient and the family. A treatment plan outline (see appendix II), developed as part of the policies and procedures for the team, helps to assure that all pertinent issues are addressed and the goals and care plan clearly delineated.

8.5 Case Revisited

In the case of Mr. Pimm, there were three stages in the evolution of his treatment plan. The first dealt with his decision to forego further radiation therapy; the second, palliative care with limits on the intensity of care as negotiated by the patient and the health care team; and third, the decisions concerning his final illness, made largely by the team under Mr. Pimm's advance directives.

The decision to discontinue radiation therapy confronts the issue of quality of life versus quantity. The treatments had rendered Mr. Pimm weak and anorexic to the point of seeking institutionalization. He was quite relieved at the prospects of the option of this course, and regained a measure of hope and joy in living which carried him through the setback of having to confront the documented metastases and inevitability of death.

In helping him to make this decision, the team also felt an obligation to the science of medicine and to the "contract" that Mr. Pimm had made with the radiation oncologist. Although patient autonomy would outweigh these factors, the team may have wished to present the importance of continuing within a research protocol. Also, should further palliative radiation become indicated, it would be to Mr. Pimm's advantage that the oncologist feel an ongoing sense of commitment to his care.

The second stage of the treatment plan is most clearly the transition from curative to palliative care. Mr. Pimm was confronted with a variety of options. These involved not only determining the extent of his treatment, but also the setting of his continued care. The health care contract becomes open for renegotiation from the standpoint of both the patient and provider. For instance, Mr. Pimm elected to remain in the facility rather than return home. By refusing intensive care, the team could effectively argue that acute hospital transfer would no longer be of benefit because of the services available to him in the hospice. He chose active treatment of intercurrent illnesses with intravenous hydration and antibiotics, yet refused long-term enteral nutritional support. Finally, he expressed his desires in the form of an advance directive should he become incompetent.

At the third stage, the realization of the terminal event, the team acted on Mr. Pimm's directive in not continuing useless treatment. An important issue revolves around the decision by the covering physician to administer a final intramuscular injection. This seemingly futile gesture should be construed as an acknowledgment of the significance of a *team* decision in withdrawing care. The process of accepting the inevitability and imminence of death helps to reconfirm each team member's commitment to care at this final stage.

8.6 Conclusion

We have argued in this chapter that the health care professional may have a moral obligation to withhold treatment, even life-sustaining treatment, for several reasons. First, and most importantly, the withholding or withdrawing of treatment may be consistent with the competently expressed wishes of the patient. The patient may base such a decision upon such factors as the quality of life or excessive costs. Withholding or withdrawing treatment under such circumstances respects the moral autonomy of the patient. Second, treatment may be withheld from the incompetent patient (with the permission of the ethically and legally appropriate parties) when doing so is consistent with a medically coherent plan to relieve patient suffering. Finally, as health care professionals, we must be aware of the increasing pressures upon the health care profession to conserve scarce and expensive societal resources.

Annotated Bibliography

Besdine RW. "Decisions to Withhold Treatment from Nursing Home Residents," *Journal of the American Geriatrics Society* 31(10): 602–06 (1984).
Besdine points out that the types of issues involved in limited treatment choices are quite different in the hospital and nursing home settings. While much of the ethics literature has focused upon the dramatic sorts of limited treatment issues common in the acute care hospital setting, less attention has been paid to the more cloudy and vexing questions raised in the long-term chronic care environment of the nursing home.
Lo B, and Jonsen AR. "Clinical Decisions to Limit Treatment," *Annals of Internal Medicine* 93:764–68 (1980).
Though this article has been treated much more thoroughly and more recently by such as the President's Commission, it still bears attention as a pioneering attempt to recognize the ethical value of limited treatment and to provide some rational criteria for choosing limited treatment options.
Miles SH. "The Limited Treatment Plan," Parts I-IV *Clinical Report on Aging* 1(1–4) (1987).
This series of short articles by Miles provides an excellent overview of the purposes and practicalities of limited treatment plans. They could be of great help for the practicing physician.

Miles SH, and Ryden MB. "Limited Treatment Policies in Long-Term Care Facilities," *Journal of the American Geriatrics Society* 33(10): 707–11 (1985).
This article surveys the development of limited treatment policies in long-term care facilities in Minnesota. The data presented by Miles and Ryden show that while progress has been made in gaining acceptance for limited treatment choices, much still needs to be done. For example, only a handful of those institutions contacted had a limited treatment policy. Furthermore, many of those policies did not allow the patient involved much of a voice in limited treatment choices.

References

American College of Physicians. *Ethics Manual*, 1984.
American Medical Association (Statement of the Council on Ethical and Judicial Affairs). "Withholding or Withdrawing Life Prolonging Medical Treatment," March 15, 1986.
Braithwaite S, and Thomasma DC. "New Guidelines on Foregoing Life-Sustaining Treatment in Incompetent Patients: An Anti-Cruelty Policy," *Annals of Internal Medicine* 104:711–15 (1986).
Callahan D. *Setting Limits,* New York: Simon and Schuster, 1987.
Cassell EJ. "The Nature of Suffering and the Goals of Medicine," *New England Journal of Medicine* 306 (11):638–45 (1982).
Hilfiker D. "Allowing the Debilitated to Die: Facing Our Ethical Choices," *New England Journal of Medicine* 308 (12):716–19 (1983).
Koop CE. "The Sanctity of Life," *Journal of the Medical Society of New Jersey* 75 (1): 62–67 (1978).
Thomasma DC. "Quality of Life Judgment, Treatment Decisions and Medical Ethics," *Clinics of Geriatric Medicine* 2:17–27 (1986).

CHAPTER 9

The Withholding or Withdrawing of Nutrition and Hydration

The Case of Aunt Audrey

"Aunt Audrey was actually the last surviving sister of our grandmother's family. A large, strong-willed woman who had never married, she instead devoted her considerable energies to the local chapters of civic associations and political groups. We only grew to appreciate her strengths when we, embroiled in our college protest marches, found an ally and compatriot amongst our parents' parents' generation.

"Because she lived near the university campus, as well as our 'spiritual' closeness, her home became a favorite meeting place of our social group at school. Even though we graduated, paired-off and began our careers and families, the attachments persisted and we visited often. When Aunt Audrey reached her late 70s, her health began to wane. Our visits grew to become as much for necessity as pleasure.

"The real problems began with a small area of gangrene on her big toe which refused to heal because of diabetes. It festered, slowly enlarged and eventually led to an amputation below the knee. This was a devastating blow to her independence and, symbolically, to her psyche. She decided to enter a nursing home after her hospitalization for what turned out to be a futile attempt at rehabilitation.

Her personality hardened and lost its edge of cynical humor; she was openly through with life.

"Life was not through with Aunt Audrey, however. She lived a tolerable existence in the nursing home for several more years. Her size and demeanor were quite intimidating, which got her what she needed, although she had no friends among "those blathering idiots"—a not-so-endearing term she used to describe nearly everyone associated with the institution. This situation continued until a stroke robbed her of the ability to move her right side or speak.

"After a brief and unrewarding hospitalization, Aunt Audrey returned to the nursing home. On her first night, she pulled out the nasogastric tube and fought the nurse who tried to reinsert it. Sedatives and restraints were ordered but she still managed to extubate herself. Finally, a family meeting was called by her physician. We were presented with the options of a gastrostomy tube, four-point restraints with heavy sedation, or syringe feedings—which she had previously refused.

"It was quite obvious to the family that Aunt Audrey was now pursuing death as single-mindedly and fervently as any cause in her life. We elected to continue syringe feedings. Although we visited often, she never acknowledged our presence. About a week later she lapsed into a coma. No attempt to rehydrate her was made and she expired in several days. The talk at her funeral revolved around her strength and refusal to be dominated by suffering."

Discussion

Of those patients who are maintained by the artificial provision of nutrition and hydration, the vast majority are elderly. The U.S. Office of Technology Assessment has pointed out (1987) that the most common causes for such intervention are eating disorders closely related to dementia. Hence, the health care professional who cares for the elderly is likely to face the prospect of either placing a patient on indefinite artificial nutrition and hydration or allowing death to occur as a natural outcome of an eating disorder.

Since the preceding chapter discussed the ethics of withholding or withdrawing medical treatments, one might ask why a separate chapter discussing ethical issues surrounding the provision of nutrition and hydration is required. The relevant difference between nutrition and hydration and other sorts of medical treatment is that nutrition and hydration are often seen not (or at least not only) as *medical treatment*, but as a fundamental expression of human caring for the patient. Withdrawing or withholding nutrition and hydration would amount to ceasing to care—the essence of the health *care* professions. The ethics of nutrition and hydration would be vastly different from other types of patient treatment.

This chapter argues that such a distinction is mistaken, and that in some circumstances it is ethically proper to withhold or withdraw nutrition and hydration. Respect for patient autonomy and the obligation to relieve suffering or to do no harm are the ethical principles which shall figure most prominently in our discussion. Before turning to the ethical aspect of this controversy, let us begin by considering what is meant by nutritional and hydrational support.

9.1 Techniques for Nutrition and Hydration

There are several ways in which a patient can receive nutritional and fluid support. For the purposes of our discussion, let us assign the various methods to three different levels of intervention.

Level I. Oral Feeding
Two types of nutritional support fall under this category:

1. Allowing the patient to feed himself.
2. Spoon feeding, as tolerated by the patient.

Both of these methods of feeding have the advantage of not forcing the patient to do anything against his or her wishes. The trouble with both methods is that if the patient is unwilling to eat (e.g., refuses to feed himself or spits out food that is spoon fed) or unable (e.g., because of being in a coma), there will be inadequate intake. Over time, if intake is inadequate, the patient will die.

Level II. Technical Intervention

Level II includes the methods available for providing nutrition and hydration when the methods of Level I do not provide adequate intake and the health care professional wants to ensure sufficient intake. These methods include:

1. Nasogastric tube: a flexible plastic tube is inserted through the nose, down the throat and into the stomach.
2. Gastrostomy: A hole is surgically created allowing access to the stomach through the abdominal wall. Liquid nutrition is pumped through a tube in the hole into the stomach.
3. Intravenous feeding: Fluids are delivered through a standard IV needle in a major vein of one of the extremities.
4. Hyperalimentation: Fluids are delivered through a large bore needle usually inserted in the subclavian vein.

Each of these methods, with the exception of intravenous feeding, can provide long-term nutritional support. There are, however, disadvantages. The nasogastric tube can be uncomfortable for many patients. Competent patients sometimes reject it, while many incompetent patients may persist in pulling the tube out. Nasogastric tubes also run the risk of irritation to the passages through which the tube passes as well as aspiration caused by regurgitation of stomach contents into the lungs. A gastrostomy (or pharyngotomy or esophagostomy) is often better tolerated by patients, but it involves a surgical procedure under anesthesia. Hence elderly patients face the risks of anesthesia, surgery, and post-surgical infections. There are the risks of aspiration, and the tube may block the pylorus, preventing the movement of stomach contents into the intestines. Intravenous feeding causes little direct suffering, but it cannot provide adequate support for long-term care, and the IV sites are subject to clotting, deterioration, and infection. Finally, hyperalimentation requires surgical placement in a major vein, which carries risks. Because it taps into a central vein, it increases the risk of significant infection.

With all-artificial feeding, since the feeding solution is nutritionally rich and dispensed over a period of time, there is significant risk of bacterial contamination, which can cause diarrhea, gastroenteritis, and bacteremia (Office of Technology Assessment, 1987).

All methods in this level, because of their invasive nature, require patient or surrogate consent.

Level III. No Feeding

Level III represents a kind of non-intervention. If the patient is unwilling or unable to eat or drink by mouth, and for some reason none of the techniques of Level II are chosen, then the patient is allowed to go without nutrition or hydration. Over time, such treatment (or non-treatment) leads to death, though the patient may actually die of some other cause before succumbing to malnutrition or dehydration.

The real ethical difficulties arise in three sorts of circumstances:

> (1) A competent patient chooses not to be subjected to Level II type interventions
> (2) An incompetent but conscious patient refuses to eat
> (3) Irreversibly comatose patients unable to eat who can only be maintained by Level II type interventions.

In section 9.3 we develop an ethical framework for approaching these issues, and in 9.4 we use that framework to consider these particular kinds of cases.

9.3 The Ethics of Nutritional and Hydrational Intervention

A variety of arguments are offered supporting the conclusion that the provision of nutrition and hydration, even if requiring Level II type intervention, is morally obligatory. Included are:

> (a) That death by dehydration and malnourishment is painful
> (b) That withdrawing or withholding nutrition and hydration is tantamount to *killing* the patient
> (c) That providing nutrition and hydration, even if it must be done artificially, is not simply medical treatment, but an expression of fundamental human caring.
> Let us consider each of these arguments in turn.

(a) That Death by Dehydration and Malnourishment Is Painful

If indeed the withholding or withdrawing of nutritional and hydrational support caused significant patient discomfort, that would count as a weighty ethical argument against such practices. In many cases, to do so to a patient could cause significant discomfort. If the patient has not autonomously chosen such a course of action, one has at least a *prima facie* ethical reason for not withholding or withdrawing such treatment.

One must be careful, however, in supposing that the patient experiences dehydration and malnourishment in the same way as an otherwise healthy person. For many elderly patients, suffering from advanced, chronic, painful, and irreversible diseases, nutritional and hydrational support may well cause more discomfort than its absence. Intervention may prolong a painful dying process. Comfort might best be achieved by frequently rinsing the patient's mouth or using ice chips to relieve the "dry mouth" sensation.

When the quality of life of an elderly patient is extremely low because of chronic pain or advanced dementia, the invasiveness of the nutritional support can be quite discomforting. Many demented patients must be restrained in order to prevent them from repeatedly pulling out feeding tubes. This should be understood as expressing at least some degree of distaste or discomfort because of the feeding tube. Furthermore, diarrhea and other bacterial infections are common side effects of such feeding methods. These lend their own discomfort and indignity to the patient. Lastly, the presence of the feeding apparatus and its entry into the patient can be a significant emotional barrier between the patient and family members, thus causing important emotional losses.

We must conclude that patient comfort is not enhanced by Level II type feeding interventions, at least in many instances.

(b) That Withdrawing or Withholding Nutrition and Hydration Is Tantamount to Killing the Patient

It can be argued that withdrawing or withholding nutrition and hydration is no different from killing the patient. We are unconvinced by this. As we showed in the preceding chapter, it can be ethically proper to withhold or withdraw certain forms of treatment even when doing so may cause death. Our argument there was that the preservation of life is not the *only* goal of medicine, and that one of its other important goals, the relief of suffering, sometimes necessitates courses of action that may shorten life. If it is ethical to withhold antibiotics, surgery, or other forms of medical treatment because the burdens outweigh the benefits to the patient, why should it not be the same for nutritional and hydrational support? This argument rests upon the claim that providing nutrition and hydration is not on a par with medical treatments. So it is to that claim that we must turn our attention.

(c) That Providing Nutrition and Hydration Is Not Simply Medical Treatment, but an Expression of Fundamental Human Caring

The core of the ethical dispute concerning the obligatoriness or non-obligatoriness of nutritional and hydrational support concerns whether such intervention is simply one of many sorts of medical "treatment" or whether it differs substantially from medical "treatment." For if it is simply another form of medical treatment, there is no special reason that food and fluids should be required for every patient. On the other hand, if such intervention does not differ in kind from other medical intervention, there seems to be no reason why food and fluids might not be withdrawn under certain circumstances, even if doing so may lead to a patient's death.

Taking the first stance, that providing nourishment and fluids is more than just treatment, the Vatican argued, for example, that:

> If the patient is in permanent coma, irreversible as far as it is possible to predict, *treatment* is not required, but *care, including feeding,* must be provided. (Pontifical Academy of Sciences, 1985, emphases added)

Clearly the Vatican considers providing nutrition and hydration not simply "treatment," but a more fundamental kind of basic care. A similar position is argued by Meilaender (1984), who states:

> If there is any way in which the living can stand by those who are not yet dead, it would seem to be through the continued provision of food and drink even when the struggle against disease has been lost. To continue to nourish the life of one who has been defeated in that battle is the last evidence we can offer that we are more than frontrunners, that we are willing to love to the very point of death.

Meilaender argues that treatment is designed to cure or heal disease. Therefore, treatment may ethically be withheld or withdrawn when cure is impossible and is no longer the aim of medical care. Food and water, on the other hand, are needed by all humans, *even when they are not ill*. To further emphasize the distinction, Meilaender argues that when we withdraw respiratory support from a patient, the patient may always surprise us by breathing on his own (as indeed happened in the Karen Quinlan case). But if we withdraw nutrition and hydration from a patient, then death will *inevitably* ensue. Therefore, food and water should not be viewed as medical *treatment*. They should be viewed as a basic sort of obligation which we have to all humans, dying or not.

Meilaender is willing to consider the possibility of withdrawing such support from conscious patients for whom life has become burdensome and for whom interventionist nutrition and hydration would be so burdensome that it is better to die (e.g., because of intense and unremitting pain caused by a terminal illness). But concerning the comatose, he insists (1984, p. 13) that:

> For the permanently unconscious person, feeding is neither useless nor excessively burdensome. It is ordinary human care and is not given as treatment for any life-threatening disease.

We agree with Micetich et al (1983) when they suggest that artificial nutrition and hydration is often supplied to patients for whom it constitutes no real benefit, not for the patient's sake, but as a "maneuver designed to appease the consciences of managing physicians and ancillary staff." This suggests to us that many physicians and associated health care professionals have a difficult time seeing how to *care* for a patient without applying medical technology, just as we saw in our discussion of limited treatment plans. Many elderly patients are burdened with invasive feeding technologies so that health care providers can feel that they have not abandoned their patient.

There may well be a moral obligation to offer food and fluids. But, contrary to the view that artificially supplied nutrition and hydration (i.e., what we have termed Level II type interventions) are some special sort of care, we agree with the view advocated by the AMA in its 1986 statement, "Withholding or Withdrawing of Life Prolonging Medical Treatment" (AMA, 1986). Therein it is explicitly stated that technologically supplied nutrition and hydration are a form of *medical treatment* and that as such they may ethically be withdrawn or withheld under the same sorts of circumstances that justify such action with regard to other sorts of medical treatment. The Massachusetts Medical Society adopted a similar policy in 1985, as did the California Medical Association in 1986. Furthermore, this is a view which has been upheld in several recent court decisions, such as: New York Supreme Court, *In re Application of Plaza Health and Rehabilitation Center,* 1984; New Jersey Supreme Court, *In re Conroy,* 1985; California District Court of Appeal, *Bouvia v. Superior Court,* 1986; Florida District, *Corbett v. D'Alessandro,* 1986; and Massachusetts Supreme Judicial Court, *Brophy v. New England Sinai Hospital,* 1986. There is, however, disagreement in these decisions concerning under what circumstances artificial nutrition and hydration may be withheld or withdrawn.

9.4 Decision Making

Since we believe that artificially supplied nutrition and hydration is ethically similar to other sorts of life-sustaining treatment interventions, we believe that decision making concerning withholding or withdrawing nutritional and hydrational support should be identical to the decision procedures outlined and defended in our discussion of limited treatment plans in general.

(1) The Competent Patient

Cases involving competent patients may arise in two ways directly and in one way indirectly. Directly, a patient may become incapable of swallowing and autonomously reject Level II type intervention. Alternatively, a patient may choose (because of poor quality-of-life considerations and bleak prospects) not to eat and also reject Level II type intervention. Indirectly, a patient might, in consultation with a physician, anticipate an incapacity to eat in the normal fashion and leave an advance directive of some sort indicating that Level II type interventions are not to be employed.

In such cases, the vast majority of ethicists, the President's Commission for the Study of Ethical Problems in Medicine (1983), several medical societies, and several court decisions all agree that the health care professional's moral obligation to respect the autonomy of patients applies in these circumstances.

One must be careful, though, to distinguish between a moral obligation not to force feed an unwilling competent patient and the right not to accede to a patient's every wish. The ethics of artificial nutrition and hydration are not universally agreed upon. Some institutions and some individual health care professionals find it morally unacceptable to cooperate in what they perceive as a patient's immoral suicide. The best solution under such circumstances is to arrange for the transfer of the patient to the care of another institution or professional which is ethically more sympathetic to the patient's wishes.

(2) The Incompetent but Conscious Patient

Despite some suggestion to the contrary (e.g., Meilaender, 1984), we believe that the decision to withhold or withdraw artificial nutrition and hydration is ethically most complex and difficult in cases involving demented patients. Though demented, these patients may often still possess a capacity to participate in life. Thus, the decision to intervene or not with Level II type support must be based upon a judgment concerning the burdens and discomforts of the intervention as opposed to the benefits of prolonged life. Since the demented patient cannot express in a clear and unequivocal voice how they perceive the burdens of intervention or the benefits of prolonged life, the judgment (barring advance directives) must be made upon the appearances of burden and benefit. As we have repeatedly argued, the difficulty of such decision making and the risk of mistaken judgment on our part should not preclude the right of incompetent patients to have treatment withheld or withdrawn.

To protect the rights of the demented patient and to ensure thoughtful decision making, these are cases especially suited for joint involvement of the health care team (especially those members involved in day-to-day care), family members (if any), and the institutional ethics committee.

(3) The Irreversibly Comatose Patient

In the case of irreversibly comatose patients, it is hard to see how Level II type intervention provides any benefit to the patient. Such intervention does nothing to "cure" the underlying medical problem; nor does it do anything to ameliorate the symptoms of permanent loss of consciousness; nor does the withholding or withdrawing of such support seem to cause any suffering. It has been pointed out (Meilaender, 1984) that Level II type interventions cannot be said to cause any pain or discomfort to the comatose patient. We suggest, however, that even if one accepts that such intervention does not cause any pain or discomfort, it is still ethically permissible to withdraw or withhold such support.

First, such intervention is *futile* (Lynn and Childress, 1983). That is, it does nothing to cure or ameliorate the underlying condition of permanent loss of consciousness. Second, since such patients are irreversibly lost to any social interaction, to prolong their biological lives would be an act of *cruelty*, in the words of Braithwaite and Thomasma (1986).

The decision to withhold or withdraw Level II type intervention should be a consensual decision involving the health care team and the patient surrogate. It may also be prudent to involve the institutional ethics committee even if the health care team and surrogate are in agreement.

9.5 Case Revisited

Aunt Audrey had clearly stated her wish not to have her life prolonged and acted on these intentions in a silent but unmistakable way. Despite the difficulties of watching her passing, the sense of defending her autonomy was equally clear and allowed the staff and "family" to bear the discomfort which we—but not she—suffered. For in fact, virtually no discomfort was ever perceived, a finding often commented upon by others and substantiated by research in the surprising lack of response to the thirst drive under these circumstances.

Problems arise when either the prior decision was not made clear or the patient was unable to "express" his wishes through action. The language of most Living Wills includes references to life-prolonging measures which would cover these eventualities; none, however, *specifically* address this point. The emotional charge often associated with nutrition and hydration makes this issue one that needs to be discussed specifically in prescribing the treatment plan. One subtle but important point is that the options were presented in the order of preference for the staff; likewise, a recommendation for life-sustaining measures should be the default position. Withdrawal of nutrition and hydration should be made an active decision by the surrogate.

Mechanical or technical difficulties should not be the deciding factor unless at the extremes, e.g., requirement for total parenteral nutrition. By the same argument, the most expeditious means of providing nutrition and hydration should be actively sought if sustenance is to be pursued.

When no prior statement is available, two behaviors usually prompt consideration for withdrawal: deep and irreversible coma and active resistance to attempts to provide sustenance. Aunt Audrey was active in her resistance, and therefore the concerns of respecting her autonomy were more obvious. This is less clear in cases of irreversible coma. The irony is that these patients generally have a worse prognosis and are more withdrawn from their environment, but are easier to manage, so the autonomy issues are not raised. We would argue that both conditions are actually related to mechanical problems and such behaviors should not play the deciding role in the decision.

The last point is that withdrawal of nutrition and hydration must not also signal withdrawal of emotional support and human contact. Under these circumstances the staff needs to be most vigilant and attentive to the other needs of the patient and family. Patients are most vulnerable to neglect and the staff most susceptible to nihilism. Refocusing the care protects both from these unwanted developments. In addition, the emotional detachment which often precedes such a consideration makes this dying different from that associated with the acute phase of the illness. Families will be more likely to need assistance with their feelings of separation and release.

9.6 Conclusion

In our view, it is ethically sensible to regard Level II type nutritional and hydrational intervention as medical treatment. The ethics of withholding or withdrawing artificial nutrition and hydration are essentially the same as other sorts of choice to limit treatment. The death of the patient following withdrawal or withholding of such support should not be seen as caused by the withdrawal or withholding of artificial support, but as a result of the chronic, underlying condition which makes normal feeding (i.e., Level I type support) unsuccessful. Elderly persons, especially the demented, should not be forced to endure the burden and indignity of permanent artificial nutrition and hydration just to assuage the feelings of the health care professional or family members. To do so would be unnecessarily cruel to the patient.

Annotated Bibliography

Meyers DW. "Legal Aspects of Withdrawing Nourishment from an Incurably Ill Patient," *Archives of Internal Medicine* 145:125–28 (1985).
  Meyers provides a concise summary of the reasoning behind the decision to withdraw or withhold artificial feeding, concluding that there are good ethical reasons for sometimes choosing to withhold or withdraw such treatment. He then provides a review of legal decisions relating to this controversy, and concludes by proposing a clear legal rationale for choosing to withhold or withdraw artificial nutrition or hydration

Office of Technology Assessment (Congress of the United States). *Life-Sustaining Technologies and the Elderly,* Washington, D.C.: US Government Printing Office, 1987.
  This important work provides a sustained assessment of the varieties and efficacies of various medical interventions for the elderly. Sections on CPR and artificial nutrition and hydration are quite good. A "Summary" version of the study is available.

References

Braithwaite S, and Thomasma DC. "New Guidelines on Foregoing Life-Sustaining Treatment in Incompetent Patients: An Anti-Cruelty Policy." *Annals of Internal Medicine* 104:711–15 (1986).

CHAPTER 10

Resuscitation

The Case of Mrs. Parrot

Mrs. Parrot had been the matriarch of her household, the pillar of her church and a respected leader of the parents' group in the local school system. As she got older, it was often remarked that hers would probably be the most well attended funeral in the neighborhood. She trusted in her doctor and in the Lord for good health, which she enjoyed until she reached her eighty-second year. And then, one morning, she didn't arise. A massive stroke had rendered her comatose. The community's outpouring of sympathy was equal to everyone's expectations. Her room at the hospital was filled with flowers and cards, well-wishers came in a steady stream and the church women kept a constant vigil with donated private-duty care. But Mrs. Parrot was not yet ready to die.

A painful realization came to her family as she lay in her bed, as the days became weeks. Not only did the attention wane, but the pressure to find alternative living arrangements became palpable. But her children had followed her lead: all had the responsibilities of careers, families, and social obligations of their own. And none could take her home.

From these ashes, the oldest daughter, Mrs. Yates, ascended to the vacated matriarchical role. She arranged for her mother to be transferred to a skilled nursing facility, and for the distribution of her possessions and liquidation of the estate.

Unfortunately, Mrs. Parrot continued to linger. Soon she developed large pressure sores and became septic. Antibiotics were administered and the ulcers were debrided—but she was too poor a candidate for plastic surgery. Her condition was obviously getting worse despite the active intervention of the staff.

Mrs. Yates never lost hope. When approached about the withdrawing of treatment in the face of impending death, Mrs. Yates demanded that everything possible be done. Another course of antibiotics and another round of debridements were ordered—to no avail.

The situation quickly deteriorated when Mrs. Parrot developed pneumonia. The organisms were especially destructive of lung tissue and resistant to antibiotic therapies. When she began to show signs of respiratory distress, Mrs. Yates insisted on hospital transfer to the ICU. She wanted her mother intubated and mechanically ventilated. She also specified that if her heart stopped, she was to be resuscitated. "She always taught me to keep faith with hope and prayer," said Mrs. Yates. "Where there's life, there's hope. I'll never give up!"

Discussion

Beginning in the 1960s, great progress was made in the technology of cardiopulmonary resuscitation (CPR). By a combination of physical massage, pharmacological stimulus, electrical stimulus, and ventilatory assistance, health care professionals acquired astonishing abilities to restore heartbeat and respiration. Enamored of this technology, the health care industry quickly expanded its application beyond its original use in treatment of post-operative arrests and emergency intervention. By the mid 1970s, it had become common institutional policy that CPR be administered to virtually any and every hospital patient suffering a cardiopulmonary arrest, whatever the patient's underlying condition. Thus, from being fairly unlikely candidates for CPR, the elderly soon became common recipients of this form of treatment.

The vastly expanded criteria for CPR included many patients who were suffering from chronic and irreversible underlying conditions which were either the cause or a contributing factor to the arrest. Not surprisingly, challenges to the ethics of such wide-spread administration of CPR began to appear.* Since then, the ethical appropriateness of "do not resuscitate" orders (DNR) has become a topic of widespread discussion. Recent ethical policy statements by the AMA, the American College of Physicians, and the President's Commission argue that, while many elderly patients are medically and ethically proper candidates for CPR, far too many have CPR unethically and unbeneficially inflicted upon them. CPR interventions provide a classic example of how we can easily become enticed to apply certain medical technologies far beyond their ethically proper domain.

For simplicity's sake, we shall structure our discussion around three ethical principles which should be familiar to the health care professional—autonomy, beneficence, and justice.

10.1 CPR and Autonomy

There are two ways in which respect for autonomy figures into DNR decisions: patient autonomy and physician autonomy.

Patient Autonomy

Under the principle of autonomy, the health care professional has a moral obligation to respect the wishes of a competent patient. This includes the patient's decision to refuse treatment, even if it is life-saving treatment. There is no reason why CPR interventions should be an exception to this rule.

Yet a research project by Bedell, Delbanco, and Cook (1984) has shown that a large percentage of physicians do not consult with their patients on this matter, *even when there is a high expectation of cardiopulmonary arrest*. Many of the physicians in the survey who refrained from discussing the matter with their patients claimed to have known what their patients' preferences were in this matter. Nevertheless, the survey of the patients involved showed that the physicians were astonishingly *inaccurate* in their claims to known their patients' preferences. To make matters worse, CPR is a kind of intervention that precludes consulting patients at the time of the event. Thus patient autonomy can only

---

*Landmark articles in this vein include: Lemire J and Johnson A, 1972; AMA, 1974; and Rabkin MT, Gillerman G, and Rice NR, 1976.

be respected by directly confronting the issue with the patient prior to the crisis. Persistent physician reluctance in this matter has led many institutions, particularly nursing homes, to require that a resuscitation status be decided upon when a patient is first admitted. This decision is, of course, open to revision and should be periodically reviewed. By clearly defining the issue and fostering patient awareness and participation, the institution promotes patient autonomy and also provides legally protecting documentation for the health care provider. Properly executed Living Wills or durable power of attorney may serve to achieve the same goals.

Respect for patient autonomy requires that the patient have a reasonably accurate understanding of the procedure in question. This means that the health care professional must provide a realistic explanation of CPR as well as its likely outcomes. Given the often brutally invasive nature of CPR and its generally poor prognosis, it is understandable that many elderly patients would rather forego the option or restrict it to specific circumstances where the physician believes there are strong indications for long-term success (e.g., where the underlying cause is acute and readily reversible). This is especially true when one understands that even when successful, resuscitation does not by itself improve the patient's quality of life over what it was before the arrest. Indeed, overall quality of life may be much less than before the arrest. It is not surprising, therefore, that many elderly decide that the risks of CPR are not commensurate with its possible benefits for their lives.

Decision making is, of course, different in the case of incompetent patients. As we have discussed elsewhere (see chapters 2 and 6), decision making for incompetent patients is best guided by advance directives or (lacking such directives) consensus between the health care team and the next of kin. Ethics committees can help resolve conflict between these parties. And in the absence of competent family members, the state may appoint a guardian. Every effort should be made to ascertain what the patient's wishes would be if he or she could speak competently. Lacking such knowledge, decision making should be guided by principles of beneficence and justice.

Physician Autonomy

Respect for patient autonomy does not entail that the health care professional must accede to a patient's every wish. The moral autonomy of the professional is of just as much moral value as the autonomy of the patient. This means that while the physician should not violate a patient's wishes concerning CPR, he or she is not bound absolutely to accommodate such wishes. The physician should, therefore, keep professional standards in mind.

Blackhall (1987) points out that it has become common practice to administer CPR to any patient in the hospital (except those who specifically refuse the option) who suffers a cardiopulmonary arrest, regardless of the underlying cause. But CPR was not developed for such a broad application and its success rate in such applications is dismally poor. As Blackhall notes, studies since 1960 have reported survival rates (e.g., hospital discharge) of 5–23 percent, with most studies reporting less than 15 percent. Since these figures represent *overall* survival rates, the likelihood of success for those who have underlying medical illnesses (such as pneumonia, sepsis, congestive heart failure) is undoubtedly very low. For instance, for cancer, it is nil; for dialysis is it around 3 percent. (See Blackhall [1987] and Bedell, Delbanco, and Cook [1983].)

Despite these unimpressive figures, CPR is sometimes desired by patients (more so by family members) either under the rubric of "do everything" or as a last desperate attempt to forestall death. This raises two ethical questions for the health care professional: (1) What are our ethical obligations when a patient or family requests CPR in circumstances where it is not "medically appropriate treatment"? (2) Do we have a moral obligation to mention the option of CPR when not specifically requested in those instances where it would not be (in our judgment) "medically appropriate treatment"?

First, let us clarify what is meant by "medically appropriate treatment" in this context. According to the American College of Physicians *Ethics Manual* (1984), medical treatment is appropriate when it is likely to "restore the patient to a state of reasonable comfort and function." By inference, CPR is not medically indicated in cases where this is not reasonable expectation. Thus, the *Ethics Manual* concludes:

> If a physician decides that the disease process or other medical condition that the patient has would not positively be affected by the initiation of resuscitative efforts—in other words, if resuscitative efforts would

> only prolong the dying process—then a decision to
> write a do-not-resuscitate order is ethically proper.

This view is shared by the AMA (1980) and the President's Commission (1983).

Returning to our first question, what are the physician's moral obligations when patients or families request medically inappropriate resuscitative measures? Suppose, for example, that while it is the physician's judgment that CPR would provide no benefit to the patient, the patient (or the incompetent patient's family or legal guardian) insists that CPR be provided. What should the physician do?

The physician does have a moral obligation to inform patients (or, when incompetent, their families) of "medically appropriate treatment" and to counsel them in their choices. There is no professional obligation to provide treatment which is inappropriate. The physician is, however, obligated to help transfer such patients, if disagreement persists after discussion, to care givers who may agree with their requests.

The second issue is whether the physician has a moral responsibility to *offer* CPR when it is not medically warranted. Most agree that physicians should not proffer treatment which poses harm to the patient and which presents little or no possibility of benefit. This is consistent with the maxim, "above all, do no harm." Although not a unanimous view (see, e.g., the President's Commission, 1983), Blackhall (1987) has concluded from the "do no harm" rule that the physician is under no moral obligation to even mention CPR as a possibility when sound medical judgment is that it would be medically inappropriate.

While such a position makes good sense, it seems to overlook the fact that, for better or worse, full CPR effort is the default status at most acute care institutions, despite the recognition that CPR is not a miraculously successful procedure and that it holds the potential to inflict much harm and suffering. No other medical treatment on a par with CPR is applied by default. The decision is almost always *when* to apply a treatment, not *when not* to do so. One may hope that sounder minds eventually prevail. In the meantime, it would seem that physicians ought to discuss the CPR option, even when it would be medically inappropriate, so that the patient (or family) may have the opportunity to remove themselves from the full CPR default status.

10.2 CPR and Beneficence

The principle of beneficence serves to remind us that medicine is practiced for the benefit of the patient. This means that medical treatment and decision making (within the framework of other moral constraints) should always be intended to improve the welfare of the patient. With respect to CPR and the elderly, this principle raises three issues.

First, recommendations by the physician to the patient (or family) should be motivated towards the patient's well being. Thus, the physician must have in mind a realistic assessment of the patient's prognosis with and without CPR. A study by Bedell, et al (1986) of 294 hospital patients revealed an overall CPR success rate of only 14 percent who were able to leave the hospital alive (of whom nearly 20 percent were in a persistent vegetative state). Further, no patient with metastatic cancer, acute stroke, sepsis, or pneumonia survived until discharge. No patient who required dialysis shortly before arrest survived until discharge. Only 3 percent of those with kidney failure survived. Although advanced age is not itself a good indicator of CPR success, when we keep in mind the typical cause of arrest in the elderly, these sorts of statistics are not encouraging.

The health care professional must accept that CPR, *per se*, will not improve the patient's condition over what it was before the arrest; it is not a form of rejuvenation, but merely an attempt to gain more time for the amelioration of underlying conditions. When no improvement can be expected realistically, deciding in favor of full CPR status is nothing but deceiving the patient or family.

Second, we must be careful to make sure that it is not our own discomfort, as health care providers, that motivates us to keep a patient on full CPR status. We should not practice self-deception because we are unwilling to admit our limitations in treatment and cure. In other words, the psychological comfort of the physician (e.g., believing he or she has done everything possible) must not be allowed to override the welfare of the patient.

And third, the physician should not be swayed to sanction a full CPR by considerations of the comfort of the family or under threat of legal action. Although, as we argued in chapter 2, the family can have legitimate interests in the care of its members, those interests should not be allowed to override patient interests in such cases.

10.3 CPR and Justice

Compared to many other technological interventions, CPR is relatively inexpensive. As the President's Commission argues, CPR should not be denied simply because of finances. Given that we have chosen to fund dialysis and organ transplantation, it would not be morally justified to deny CPR *to a patient who could probably benefit from it* on financial grounds.

10.4 Understanding Patient Motivations for Inappropriate CPR

As noted above, the physician has an obligation to counsel patients concerning appropriate medical treatment. As part of that counseling, the physician should make an effort to ascertain what motivates the patient (or family) to insist upon inappropriate treatment. There are two things which might motivate patients or family members to request CPR status in this kind of situation. The physician must first ascertain which reason moves his patient or family and then deal with the issue at hand.

One motivation is unrealistic expectations of CPR or ignorance of how much suffering and harm CPR may uselessly inflict upon the patient. The best resolution in these kinds of cases is patient or family education, for if their wishes are based upon a misunderstanding or misconception of CPR and its probable outcomes, education may well resolve the disagreement between the health care provider and the patient or family.

A second motivation is denial. It seems that family members in particular may seek to deny to themselves the prospect of impending and inevitable death of a beloved relative. The insistence on resuscitation, even when medical facts indicate that such intervention will not restore the patient to any reasonable sense of well being, can be a grasping at any way of avoiding reconciliation with death. The best resolution in this kind of case is recognizing and meeting the psychological needs of the patient and family in a way that assists them to recognize the futility of resuscitative measures.

If the health care team finds it impossible to gain consent to a DNR order even after trying to deal with the patient or family in the ways mentioned above, and where the team thinks it would be morally wrong to initiate CPR, the team may consider transferring care of the patient to other health care providers (providing, of course, this is done in such a way as not to abandon the patient).

10.5 Slow Codes

When faced with the choice between classifying a patient as "code" or "no code," some medical staff try instead to leap through the horns of the dilemma by running a "slow" or "limited" code. Some relevant distinctions and some reflection show, we believe, that "slow codes" are really only a way of avoiding one's moral obligation to reach a coherent decision concerning treatment options.

The decision to run a "slow code" suggests to the medical staff that while they do have a legal obligation to initiate resuscitative efforts, often because DNR orders have not been written, procedures will be begun substantially less quickly and, perhaps, will be less vigorous than in cases of a full resuscitation effort.

There is no good medical rationale for this approach. To begin with, the success of resuscitation is tied closely to both the speed and vigor with which resuscitative efforts are initiated. Furthermore, a half-hearted effort is more likely to result in a poor outcome should the patient survive. Nor is there any good legal justification for a slow code. Indeed, slow codes are a slipshod practice which raise legal and ethical questions of professional competency and patient neglect. Deciding whether a patient should be on a code or no code status can be a very difficult and time consuming decision, involving discussion with patients or families which can be awkward and troubling. Opting for a slow code cannot, however, be a justification·for avoiding decision making. For these reasons, slow codes are to be discouraged.

10.6 Limited Codes

A better approach to that middle ground between a DNR order and a full resuscitation code is the "limited code." By the term "limited code," we mean a treatment choice which might include some sorts of intervention but not others. For example, a patient might agree with the physician that medical intervention such as cardioversion and "basic" resuscitative procedures such as external cardiac massage should be used, but only for a specified time, and that no intubation would be permitted (Lo and Steinbrook 1983, 1563).

There are many options for limited codes here. As examples, we offer four levels of intervention:

(1) Chemical code—intravenous medication and external cardiac massage are administered to treat cardiac arhythymias and congestive heart failure
(2) Electro-chemical code—as above, but cardioversion is applied for treatment of ventricular fibrillation
(3) Intubation without extended ventilator support—as above with intubation, but if spontaneous breathing is not restored in a short (specified) time the effort is stopped
(4) Full code—as above with mechanical ventilation, pacemaker insertion and aortic balloons as indicated.

The first two options may also be time limited. For example, if there is no response within four minutes, the code is discontinued, since significant organ damage is more likely afterwards. Also, the code might be restricted to arrests that are witnessed. If the patient is found dead, then the code is not called since the risk of significant organ damage is quite high.

Such limited codes are a kind of limited treatment plan, and as we argued in chapter 8, limited treatment plans can make a great deal of medical and ethical sense. Designing a limited code can allow the patient some voice in treatment options, permitting them to have the advantages of certain techniques while avoiding those techniques or interventions to which they are adverse. However, in opting for a limited code, one must make certain that the patient, family, and medical staff all understand the scope of the planned intervention and that they understand the medical and ethical rationale which justifies that choice for the particular patient involved.

10.6 Case Revisited

The conflict in this case stems from a sense of futility on the part of the treating team in opposition to the daughter's dependence on hope and prayer to the *exclusion* of the team's concerns. Both are working in the context of their own beliefs in the determining factors of Mrs. Parrot's life. The team lost faith in their ability to promote the patient's well-being and see their efforts as prolonging the dying process. Mrs. Yates has been rewarded in her faith in that her mother continues to live despite the pessimism of the health care team and the weight of medical knowledge which supports their side. It is now largely her faith and determination that sustain her mother—and these must not waiver! Her insistence on the escalation of technological intervention was based on her firm conviction that if given sufficient time and depth of prayer, the miracle bringing her mother back to health would come.

The resolution came through an outside facilitator—Mrs. Yates' pastor, who effectively argued that death was the Lord's way of bringing his children home and that having lived a good life Mrs. Parrot's road to heaven was surely well paved. By continuing her prayers, she was fighting the Lord's will—not the doctor's. Within this context, the efforts by the staff were of little import and they were allowed their wishes to withdraw therapy. Mrs. Parrot "went home" shortly thereafter.

When finally analyzed, CPR as a technical issue was irrelevant, a finding which is often the case. The team's attempts to convince Mrs. Yates of their view by graphic descriptions of the resuscitative procedures and life on a respirator fell on deaf ears. They were not communicating in terms that had meaning to her concept of the situation. Their arguments were reduced to childish scare tactics.

In discussions of CPR, the importance of reaching a timely resolution is often overshadowed by the need to be complete and deliberate. Unfortunately, the delay in resolving these disagreements also affected Mrs. Parrot, who was denied a "good and timely death." Instead of a funeral service brimming with her social friends showing their admiration and respect for her long and fruitful life, her funeral was small and short. The celebration of her successes and achievements had become dulled and dimmed over the course of her protracted illness. The community had already begun to move along, putting their grieving and memories behind them.

10.7 Conclusion

The difficulties in reaching CPR decisions rarely arise from an unclear medical prognosis. They are usually motivated by unrealistic expectations of CPR on the part of physicians, patients, or families or by the inability of physicians, patient, or family to reconcile themselves to the impending death. Elderly patients—more often than physicians or patient's families are willing to give them credit for—are accepting of their late stage in life. A frank and realistic discussion between physician and patient of the merits and demerits of CPR relative to their particular physical condition is often a great help in resolving the issue. It is a discussion which the physician, on the basis of respect for autonomy, owes the patient.

Annotated Bibliography

Annas, GJ. "CPR: When the Beat Should Stop," *Hastings Center Report* 12 (5): 30–31 (1982).
 In this early article on CPR decisions, Annas argues that there are basically two sorts of reasons for deciding on a DNR status. One reason is poor medical indications, in which case, he argues, the decision should be regarded a medical decision and be made by the physician. The second is a quality-of-life consideration, and a DNR choice based upon that kind of reason should, according to Annas, be based upon patient preferences.

Bedell SE, and Delbanco TL. "Choices About Cardiopulmonary Resuscitation in the Hospital," *New England Journal of Medicine* 310(17):1089–92 (1984).
 In this seminal article, Bedell and Delbanco document, through a limited study, just how seldom physicians discuss prospective CPR status with their patients. It also documents just how dismally inaccurate physicians are in predicting what their patients' wishes are concerning CPR status.

Bedell SE, Delbanco TL, Cook F, et al. "Survival After Cardiopulmonary Resuscitation in the Hospital," *New England Journal of Medicine* 309:569–76 (1983).
 This article reviews the very low success rate for CPR in terms of leaving the hospital alive.

President's Commission for the Study of Ethical Problems in Medicine and Biomedical and Behavioral Research. *Deciding to Forego Life-Sustaining Treatment*, Washington, D.C.: U.S. Government Printing Office, 1983.
 This volume of the Commission's work devotes considerable attention to DNR decisions. Along with defining an ethical rationale for making DNR decisions, the volume includes an appendix containing model DNR policies from a variety of health care institutions.

References

American College of Physicians. *Ethics Manual,* 1984.

American Medical Association. "Standards and Guidelines for Cardiopulmonary Resuscitation and Emergency Cardiac Care," *JAMA* 244:453–509 (1980).

Bedell SE, Pelle D, Maher PL, and Cleary PD. "Do-not-resuscitate Orders for Critically Ill Patients in the Hospital: How Are They Used and What Is Their Impact"? *JAMA* 256:233–37 (1986).

Blackhall LJ. "Must We Always Use CPR?" *New England Journal of Medicine* 317(20):1281–85 (1987).

CHAPTER 11

Suicide and Euthanasia

The Case of Tammy and Dr. Bahn

"Tammy was the director of social work at our nursing home. She had reached the age of retirement some time ago, but since she was widowed and without children, there was little attraction in staying home. Besides, she was very good in her job—a true labor of love—and everyone dreaded her eventual departure. Few knew of her breast cancer, which had been diagnosed nearly eight years previously.

"The first sign of recurrence was a solitary lung mass found on a routine chest x-ray. There being no other signs of metastases, she agreed to an open lung biopsy which confirmed recrudescence of disease; all the adjacent nodes were negative. Her oncologist elected to watch her course, as there was nothing definite to treat. One year later, she developed shingles. She came to me for symptomatic relief—not wanting to 'trouble' her oncologist. I encouraged her to have a repeat bone scan, which indeed showed widespread bone involvement. The discomfort which developed shortly thereafter finally forced her to take a leave of absence.

"Tammy elected to pursue a research protocol at the university hospital, not so much from desperation as from a wish to make a final 'gift' toward medical research. Unfortunately, she did not respond and was withdrawn from the study. The pain was brought under control but the extensive pulmonary metastases were now causing her shortness of breath with minimal activity. She elected to retire but arranged her own hospice services from the staff at our hospital. I was asked to be her physician.

"A hospice team meeting was scheduled at Tammy's house—where I met her new husband! Mike and she had been living together for several years and decided to get married shortly after her lung surgery. I was asked to stay after the others had left to discuss a 'very important matter': Tammy's mother had developed breast cancer, and two years before she had planned and carried out her own suicide (in accordance with literature acquired from the American Hemlock Society). Knowing of her daughter's situation, she bequeathed these books to Tammy. Like her mother, Tammy wished to have this option available. In payment for my cooperation, she would leave these books to me.

"The discussion of Tammy's mode of dying, both naturally and by suicide, was open and frank—she had joined on my side of these talks with terminally ill patients on many occasions in the past. Mike was fully aware of his wife's decision and reconfirmed his commitment. She had read of the various methods and opted for an overdose of barbiturates. To protect me from possible incrimination, she suggested that the lethal dose be prescribed over two prescriptions, which would be filled at different pharmacies. I agreed. However, I declined the gift of the literature.

"Tammy lived another three months. The last few weeks were rather uncomfortable, more from breathlessness than pain. The day before she died, I visited her at home; Tammy was barely aware of her surroundings and I wasn't sure she recognized me. Death came while she and Mike were listening to music they had chosen for their wedding."

Discussion

11.1 Introduction

As a group, the elderly commit suicide far more than those of any other age bracket. A 1981 study revealed that although the elderly comprised 11 percent of the population, they accounted for 25 percent of all suicides (Barnes R, Keith RC, and Raskind MA, 1981). The ways in which a health care professional may become involved are varied: (1) suspicions of suicidal thinking in a patient, (2) information from a patient on his or her intentions, (3) an open or thinly-veiled request by a patient to sanction or supply the means for suicide, or (4) a request for active participation. This is an issue with which the health care professional caring for the aged must be professionally, ethically, and emotionally equipped to manage.

11.2 Terminology

Suicide is generally understood as the active taking of one's own life. Motives may vary: a desire to preserve one's honor, to escape unavoidable and irreversible pain or debility, to be relieved of a burdensome existence. *Assisted suicide* is the act of helping someone to commit suicide. This might be done by providing information on how to commit suicide with the intent of helping the individual perform the act or by providing the means (such as lethal drugs). *Euthanasia* is a term borrowed from Greek, meaning "a good death" or "dying well." *Active euthanasia,* also known as *mercy killing,* is generally understood as meaning the killing of another person, perhaps at his own request. This crosses the boundary from assisted suicide to active euthanasia because the health care professional actually performs the fatal action. This chapter focuses upon the health care professional's role in assisting suicide or participating in active euthanasia. We shall restrict the issue to those cases where three conditions hold:

(1) The patient is (or will be) suffering great pain conjoined with a terminal illness where the suffering cannot be controlled effectively by medical management.

(2) The patient autonomously chooses this course of action and is reasonable, firm and persistent in that choice.

(3) The patient is not unduly influenced by any external pressures.

11.3 Degrees of Intervention

Though it is rarely noted, one must recognize that there are degrees of involvement in assisted suicide and active euthanasia.
This is important since the professional who finds discomfort
with overt involvement may be comfortable with lesser degrees of
intervention, although the end result is the same.

1. Patient Seeking Acceptance
   On occasion, elderly patients simply want to tell
   someone about their desire or intention to commit
   suicide. All that is sought from the professional is
   some indication that this would not be morally hor-
   rendous and to accept that intention as permissible.
2. Patient Seeking Information
   At this level, the patient is seeking information on
   how to best commit suicide—which method is least
   painful, most reliable, and best for those persons left
   behind. The health care professional is a logical person from whom to seek such information.
3. Patient Seeking the Means
   The physician might be asked, for example, to prescribe fatal quantities of barbiturates or narcotics to
   commit suicide neatly and painlessly. This is clearly
   (though almost certainly legally unprovable) assisted
   suicide.
4. Active Euthanasia
   The patient desires death by intervention, yet no
   longer has the physical ability to commit suicide. The
   health care provider might be asked, for example, to
   administer a lethal injection.

11.4 Legal Issues

The law speaks clearly. It is, in almost every jurisdiction in the U.S.
and most other modern societies, illegal to either assist in a suicide
or to participate in active euthanasia. Nevertheless, physicians are
rarely charged, and in the extremely few cases which are brought
to court they have always been acquitted.

Legality or illegality, however, does not necessarily settle the
ethical issue. As we are all well aware, though we may prefer that
law mirror morality, such is not always the case. Indeed, the lack

of aggressiveness on the part of prosecutors indicates reservations on their part concerning the morality of such legislation

11.5 Ethical Arguments Concerning Assisting Suicide and Passive Euthanasia

Assisted suicide and active euthanasia are topics with which the vast majority of health care professionals feel quite uncomfortable. The Hippocratic Oath, one of the earliest documents in medical ethics, states that, "I will neither give a deadly drug to anybody if asked for it, nor will I make a suggestion to this effect." Our culture has been traditionally opposed to suicide or active euthanasia. Yet this has not always been the case, even in western society. Among the ancient Greeks, suicide and active euthanasia (even infanticide) were widely tolerated. Among the Romans, particularly the Stoic philosophers (Epictetus, Seneca, and Cicero), suicide could be morally noble. The Hippocratic School held a minority view on this matter. Even in our own time, parts of the Hippocratic Oath run counter to commonly accepted medical practices (e.g., the Oath forbids physicians to perform abortions or to perform surgery).

Western societies adopted strong prohibitions against such practices as the Christian traditions came to dominate western culture. Various religious arguments have been given against suicide and active euthanasia, including:

(1) Our lives do not belong to us, they belong to God. Hence, such acts dispose of property which does not belong to us.
(2) God forbids killing.
(3) The bearing of suffering serves a good purpose, according to God's design.

Because of these beliefs, our culture has chosen to give the anti-suicide stance of the Hippocratic Oath far wider currency than it had in its own ancient Greece.

These religious arguments remain unconvincing, however, to those who either have different religious interpretations or who subscribe to no religion. In a society such as ours, which accepts a wide variety of moral and religious beliefs, many people will be unswayed by such appeals to religious texts. Appeal must be made to arguments based upon the common denominator of reason.

As a profession which considers itself devoted to saving or bettering life (the traditional conception of medical practice), the thought of participating in the ending of life is psychologically disturbing, even repellent. Yet current mainstream conceptions of the ethical obligations of heath care professionals to respect the autonomy of their patients and to act beneficiently towards them are consistent with assisting in suicide or participating in active euthanasia under certain circumstances. Arguments invoking the principle of justice are less clear, but they still seem to weigh in favor of the moral permissibility of assisted suicide and active euthanasia.

Autonomy

As recognized by Meier and Cassel (1983), the widely agreed-upon duty to respect patient autonomy implies a moral duty to respect the patient's wishes in the matters of chosen death. As they write (p. 295):

> Proponents of active euthanasia believe that persons should be able to determine how and when they die, and that if they need assistance, the physician, although not legally obligated, may be morally justified in providing it. This argument is based on an assumption of the supremacy of human dignity, free will, and the exercise of choice.

The principle of respect for autonomy does not say that we must respect a patient's autonomy only when we agree with the choice. We should respect the autonomy of others even when we disagree with their choices. However, the principle of autonomy is qualified by the principle of justice. We need not, and should not, cooperate with the wishes of an autonomous agent when doing so unjustly harms another. For example, we should not cooperate in someone's plan to murder another person. But in many cases, (a) there are no such victims and (b) preventing suicide or euthanasia would only postpone the inevitable death a short time. Therefore, respect for the principle of autonomy entails that (at least in some cases) it would be morally permissible to assist a patient in suicide or participate in active euthanasia.

As stated, though, health care providers are not strictly obligated to provide care which runs counter to their own deeply held moral convictions. Health care professionals who for religious or other reasons find assisted suicide or active euthanasia morally reprehensible should not feel obligated to accede to their patients' wishes. They do, however, have an obligation to help transfer such patients to the care of a physician who is willing to take on this role.

It is commonly accepted that patients have the moral right to refuse life-saving treatment intervention. Physicians have the moral obligation, under appropriate circumstances, to cooperate with such requests by withholding or withdrawing treatment. We believe that by analogy the same holds true for assisted suicide and active euthanasia.

A moral duty to respect patient autonomy, therefore, seems to render assisted suicide or active euthanasia morally permissible under certain circumstances.

Beneficence and Non-Maleficence

Especially in the elderly population, the suffering which gives them the courage to broach these matters with a health care professional arises from chronic, overpowering and irreversible physical and social conditions which are beyond the ability of the physician to cure. We cannot restore the vigor and independence lost by debilitating illness. We cannot restore the long-beloved spouse lost to death. Unless one somehow sees suffering as a virtue in itself, the moral duty of beneficence can be seen as sanctioning the health care professional's participation in assisted suicide or active euthanasia, for such intervention may be the only way possible to relieve the patient of chronic, burdensome, and irreversible suffering.

It may be argued that the principle of non-maleficence prohibits physicians or other health care professionals from such activity. Indeed, the official policy of the AMA is against assisted suicide or active euthanasia. In its policy statement, "The Physician and the Dying Patient" (1973), the AMA states that, "The intentional termination of the life of one human being by another— mercy killing—is contrary to that for which the medical profession stands and is contrary to the policy of the American Medical Association." This argument is also endorsed by Jonsen, Siegler, and Winslade (1982).

Such a position, however, rests upon confused logic. It is accepted that in some cases the principle of beneficence dictates that we accede to a patient's wish to withhold or withdraw treatment because forcing treatment would only prolong suffering. In other words, the principle of beneficence obligates us to let the patient die. Having made this concession, it is then argued that the principle of non-maleficence states, "above all, do no harm." It is (presumably) a harm to kill a patient. Therefore, one may never assist in suicide or participate in active euthanasia. The obvious flaw in this argument is that while admitting the patient would suffer less by dying sooner, one at the same time holds that it would be a harm to the patient to die sooner. This is inconsistent. We ought to conclude that the principle of beneficence (consistent with the principle of non-maleficence) permits assisting in suicide or participating in active euthanasia when doing so is the only means of relieving the unbearable suffering of the patient.

Principle of Justice

The relationship between the health care professional and the patient is always set within the larger context of society. This is most often acknowledged when discussion is raised concerning the allocation of resources. It must also be considered when the moral tone of clinical decision making can effect adversely the relationship between the profession and the public at large. The bonds of trust which tie the patient-provider relationship are, in part, founded upon the belief that health care professions are committed to the preservation of life. Therefore, great care is necessary in any modification or development of exceptions to this commitment.

To put the argument in a philosophical context, some people evaluate the justice of an act according to the happiness promoted or the suffering alleviated by that *particular act*. This is called *act utilitarianism*. From the act utilitarian point of view, the health care professional's participation in assisted suicide or active euthanasia would be ethically proper when doing so would relieve burdensome, chronic, and irreversible suffering. In the case of many of the dying elderly, these conditions would be fulfilled. Thus, act utilitarianism would approve of assisted suicide or active euthanasia in many cases.

Rule utilitarianism, contrary to *act utilitarianism*, points out that our actions are always done in the broader context of society, and that breaking ordinary moral rules, though perhaps for the best in specific instances, encourages other persons to break the rules as well. Therefore, the rule utilitarian concludes that we ought to settle upon a *set of rules* which maximizes general happiness rather than treating each case on an individual basis.

Using this rule utilitarian reasoning, some persons argue that we should never assist in suicide or participate in active euthanasia even though not doing so may cause unnecessary and pointless suffering. If the public became aware that physicians were taking part in the taking of life, the bond of therapeutic trust between the health profession and society would be broken. This lack of trust would have a detrimental effect upon health care. By participating in the taking of life, we would actually be harming our patients on the whole.

We have repeatedly argued that we must place less emphasis upon the profession's mission to heal or cure and greater stress upon our obligations to relieve suffering and provide comfort, especially concerning health care for the terminally ill elderly. Longevity, without any acknowledgment of quality-of-life considerations, is not necessarily a desirable goal. The health care professional who has the moral courage to intervene in cases where the individual patient repeatedly seeks assistance and where death is clearly the *only* feasible way of relieving the patient's great suffering will, we think, earn the moral respect and admiration of his or her elderly patients. Even if we accept rule utilitarianism, one may argue that the *rules* should be changed, since assisted suicide and active euthanasia will actually increase happiness and relieve suffering in the long run. At the same time, the health profession must be careful to avoid sending the message that human life no longer has moral value. Assisted suicide and active euthanasia must only be practiced *because* of the moral value of human life.

Though we think this conclusion consistent with the principles of medical ethics, it is certain to be controversial. The understanding of the ethical role of the health care professional is in transition. The age of patient autonomy did not arrive overnight. Likewise, there will be lingering psychological discomfort with the idea of health care professionals as not only promoters of health but also as the relievers of suffering at the end of life.

A solution is needed that acknowledges the moral appropriateness of some instances of active intervention by the health care professional while recognizing the potential adverse reactions by other patients or prospective patients. We suggest that health care professionals assist in suicide or participate in active euthanasia in cases where the burden of life is overwhelming and otherwise not amenable to palliation and only for patients who display firm and durable resolve in their desire to end their suffering (and *never* against a patient's will). We also suggest that they actively seek to educate the public that such behavior is consistent with patient autonomy and beneficence and non-maleficence. Furthermore, *it is not patient abandonment* or callousness on the part of the physician. While strictly illegal, we think such actions may be morally permissible and, in many cases, morally admirable.

11.6 Conclusion

While we admit that neither the health care profession on the whole nor society at large are yet comfortable with the idea of active physician participation in the voluntary ending of life, we believe that such actions may, under certain circumstances, be morally permissible. Those conditions are: (1) death would benefit the patient, (2) the patient competently and consistently chooses this intervention, and (3) there is no external pressure upon the patient to make this choice. The age bracket of the population which most frequently manifests those circumstances is the elderly. Thus, as our elderly population increases in both numbers and advanced age, both the health care profession and society must come to grips with this issue. We hope, for the reasons brought forward in this chapter, that we move in a direction of more ethical permissiveness in this area.

Permutations

1. Suppose an elderly patient is suffering from a terminal, irreversible, and terribly painful disease, yet the patient has not broached the subject of suicide or euthanasia with the physician. Should the physician initiate discussion of these possibilities?

Normally, it is the physician's moral and professional obligations to broach with patients treatment that might be for their benefit. The basis of this obligation is the ability of the physician, because of his or her special and extensive medical training, to know ways of helping patients that they themselves may not be aware of. For example, the typical patient will not be knowledgeable enough to know the different possible treatments for an oat-cell carcinoma. It is the physician's *special* knowledge and training which creates an obligation to explain possible treatments. But in the case of suicide or euthanasia, it does not take special medical training to know that these are possible options, though medical training may be helpful in choosing how best to do it. Since the lay person can be expected to know of this option (if not know how), the physician is not under any moral obligation as a professional to broach the option. This is something best left to the patient's initiative.

> 2. Suppose that Tammy's husband rather than Tammy herself had approached the physician while Tammy was still competent. What should be done?

Significant treatment should never be administered to a competent patient without the consent of the patient. This kind of intervention, above all others, should *never* be done without the clear, firm, and consistent consent of the patient. Dr. Bahn should refuse to accede to the wishes of the husband and should clearly state that if the issue is even to be discussed it must be at the insistence of Tammy.

> 3. Suppose that the patient is incompetent, perhaps comatose, appears to be suffering and the designated legal guardian requests that the physician participate in active euthanasia for the patient's own good.

The only circumstance where we think it might be plausible for the physician to cooperate in a case like this is when (a) the patient is suffering, and (b) the patient, when competent, left advance directives explicitly authorizing such intervention under the circumstances envisaged.

Annotated Bibliography

Battin MP. "Choosing the Time to Die: The Ethics and Economics of Suicide in Old Age," pp. 161–89 in *Ethical Dimensions of Geriatric Care,* (ed. by SF Spicker, SR Ingman and IR Lawson) Boston: D. Reidel Publishing, 1987.
While acknowledging the undesirable but potential consequence of creating pressure upon some unwilling elderly persons to choose suicide or active euthanasia, Battin argues that our society ought to permit assisted suicide and voluntary ac-

tive euthanasia. Though this policy would not be age-specific, those persons who would fall within the policy would be predominantly the elderly.

Meier DE, and Cassel CK. "Euthanasia in Old Age: A Case Study and Ethical Analysis," *Journal of the American Geriatric Society* 31(5): 294–98 (1983).

Meier and Cassel explore the ethics of individual acts of assisted suicide or active euthanasia and contrast them with the ethics of social policy decisions concerning assisted suicide and active euthanasia. They argue that while isolated acts of assisted suicide or active euthanasia may be morally permissible from the point of view of the physician caring for a particular patient, a social policy making assisted suicide or active euthanasia morally and legally permissible should not be viewed as ethically desirable because of its damage to the image of the medical profession and the mistrust that it might arouse toward physicians.

Pence GE. "Do Not Go Slowly into That Dark Night: Mercy Killing in Holland," *American Journal of Medicine* 84:139–41 (1988).

Reports on the Dutch experience in allowing physicians to participate in assisted suicide and active euthanasia on behalf of their patients. It outlines current Dutch policy and the debate which it has sparked.

Rachels J. "Euthanasia," in *Matters of Life and Death*, (ed. by T. Regan), New York: Random House, 1980.

A sustained argument in favor of the moral appropriateness of active euthanasia and a suggestion on how to change current law to permit active euthanasia.

References

American Medical Association, House of Delegates. December 4, 1973.

Barnes R, Keith RC, and Raskind MA. "Depression in Older Persons: Diagnosis and Management," *Western Journal of Medicine* 153:463 (1981).

Jonsen AR, Siegler M, and Winslade WJ. *Clinical Ethics,* New York: Macmillan Publishing Co., 1982.

Meier DE, and Cassel CK. "Euthanasia in Old Age: A Case Study and Ethical Analysis," *Journal of the American Geriatric Society* 31(5): 294–98 (1983).

Rachels J. "Euthanasia," in *Matters of Life and Death*, (ed, by T. Regan) New York: Random House, 1980.

Part III

Determining the Appropriate Locus of Patient Care

CHAPTER 12

The Hospital

The Case of Mr. and Mrs. Clark

"They were an elderly couple who lived near the office. Mrs. Clark was the first to join our practice for care of her osteoarthritis and mild hypertension, but we were soon asked to see her husband as well. Mr. Clark had retired from a middle management position at the gas and electric company ten years ago and was now essentially housebound due to his failing eyesight, encroaching deafness and debilitation arthritis.

"It had only been a year since he was last seen, but the changes were obvious. Mr. Clark had lost nearly 30 pounds and was emaciated. I offered to proceed with a diagnostic evaluation as an outpatient and we agreed to seek only reversible causes of his condition. A review of symptoms revealed a mild breathlessness and a persistent cough; chest x-ray showed evidence of tuberculosis exposure but no active disease and the PPD was negative. Before the diagnostic evaluation had gone far, his condition deteriorated with signs of pneumonia.

"Mr. Clark and his family acceded to hospitalization but refused any resuscitative efforts. The children were also clear that they respected their father's readiness for death and were especially leery of a loss of control over his course within the hospital. Still, they were willing to give me a chance to find a remediable cause of his recent decline.

"He was started on broad spectrum antibiotics, but

showed no improvement in his clinical status. I began to suspect a recrudescence of TB missed by the pre-admission screening tests. An extensive radiologic and bacteriologic work-up proved negative, although I was not satisfied with the sputum samples sent for study. He refused bronchoscopy, stating that it was more invasive than we had bargained for. Then, while in the radiology department for a routine follow-up chest x-ray, Mr. Clark experienced a respiratory arrest. He was promptly intubated and his breathing assisted via an ambu bag. The radiologist then noted his no CPR status and called me in the office. I asked him to suction the lungs thoroughly and collect sputum for both routine cultures and further tuberculosis studies. He was then to transfer Mr. Clark to his room, where I would remove the endotracheal tube. Mr. Clark resumed spontaneous respirations, but not consciousness.

"His wife and family were understandably very angry about the mistaken resuscitation. They refused further tests and insisted that he be allowed to die in peace. The diagnostic studies remained inconclusive, so I stopped the antibiotics. Without a clear-cut diagnosis and without permission to pursue an etiology, I had little more to offer. And so the long vigil began.

"At first the residents were circumspect, then the lack of activity over the next few days caused their interest to wane and they asked to withdraw from the case—'There's nothing we're doing—he's just taking up a bed.' Even the nursing staff expressed their frustration and disapproval that no nourishment was being offered nor medications given. A utilization review sticker appeared in the progress notes stating that the lack of diagnostic and therapeutic intervention would soon jeopardize his acute status and that the family was at risk of responsibility for payment—'They had better not charge us for this—it's the hospital's fault!'

"It took longer than I had hoped, but I felt it was both improper and imprudent to transfer him to another facility for his last few days. After nearly a week and a half, he died quietly with his wife and family at the bedside. Yet, somehow, it was not a 'good death.'"

Discussion

Parts I and II of this study have focused upon the patient-provider relationship in terms of the individuals involved. As we have at times intimated, however, the patient-provider relationship does not exist in a vacuum. Rather, it is situated within a context. This can be ethically significant, inasmuch as the context of health care delivery can influence, and even sometimes direct, decision making concerning medical care. In this and the following two chapters, we explore how the context of three different settings of health care delivery—the hospital, the long-term care facility, and the home—are factors in medical decision making.

We have seen how the patient and the health care professional both come to the patient-provider relationship with certain values, goals, and needs or purposes. Each of these factors are elements in ethical decision making concerning medical care. In an analogous fashion, institutions have certain values, goals, and needs or purposes. A Catholic hospital, for example, operates under a different value system than a public hospital. Less explicitly, a nursing home stands for different values, goals, and needs or purposes than an acute care hospital.

One obvious sense in which institutions can have values is by their religious affiliation. Less obvious, but equally important, is that they can have values based upon what kind of medical care they focus upon. Acute care hospitals, as we shall argue, by their very nature value life and life-preserving intervention. Thus they have the goal of saving life through sophisticated medical technology. And given these values and goals, they have a need or purpose to take care of patients who make use of their technology for preserving life. As a different example, a hospice stands for very different things than the acute care hospital. Saving or preserving life is not one of its values. Instead, the hospice values patient comfort rather than cure. Its goal is to use psycho-social counseling and provide medical palliation in order to comfort patients, relieve their suffering, and help them prepare themselves for approaching death. The home, on the other hand, if we think of it as a setting of care, values the patient's independence.

The varying natures of these contexts also means that the provider and patient occupy different roles in the different settings. For example, while the physician might be the dominant figure in the hospital setting while the patient tends to be disoriented and in an alien environment, the home is certainly the "home turf" of the patient.

Just as patients can be mismatched with health care professionals who do not share their values, goals, and needs or purposes, to the ethical discomfort and dissatisfaction of all involved, patients and providers can be mismatched with institutions. The elderly patient suffering from an irreversible illness who desires only palliative care can find himself in an acute care hospital, an institution which is geared towards intervention. This can happen in two ways. First, by *poor planning* on the part of the patient and health care professionals, the patient can find himself in a setting that does not share his values, goals, and needs and purposes. A second way this can happen is through *unforeseen events* which alter the status of the patient such that what might have been a good patient-institution match ceases to be so.

Our purpose in these chapters is twofold. First, by exploring the natures of these different health care contexts, the reader may be better equipped to recognize the potential for patient-institution mismatch. And second, having recognized what these mismatches might be, the reader will become more adept at avoiding or minimizing patient-institution mismatch. If this can be done, then the health care professional will face far fewer ethical conflicts between obligations to the patient versus those to the institution.

12.1 The Hospital Setting

As we have noted, hospitals may have their values framed by a religious or public mission. Hospitals with religious affiliations such as Catholic or Lutheran are guided by the ethical values of their sponsoring church denomination. In choosing a locus for health care delivery, both patient and provider should keep this in mind. Public and community hospitals, on the other hand, have some of their values set by the community mandate which governs them. This mandate may include, for example, a special obligation to provide health care for the poor. What most concerns us in this chapter, however, is the special values that acute care hospitals have simply by being acute care institutions. While this is not an issue of medical ethics which is exclusively an issue of geriatric medicine, the potential for patient-hospital mismatch of values and goals seems greatest among care for the elderly.

Values: In addition to having its value commitments as a religious-affiliated hospital, a public hospital, a teaching hospital, etc., the acute care hospital is based in general upon the value of promoting life. The patient who dies is seen by the institution as a lost battle. The acute care hospital setting, therefore, values the patient who wants to live, who wants to be saved by the institution.

Goals: The acute care hospital expresses its value of saving life through its medically sophisticated intervention in the lives of patients. It is chiefly concerned with serious, life-threatening illness which requires medical intervention. That intervention is characterized by its use of highly sophisticated medical technology. It is the setting of technologically supported diagnosis, such as CTscans, and of subsequent highly technological medical treatment.

Needs or Purposes: If the acute care facility is to continue to carry out its mission of providing highly technological medical care for the purposes of saving lives, at least two things must be true. First, it must have patients who want and need just that kind of care. And second, since the provision of the technology to support such care is an expensive proposition, the hospital must frequently use its equipment. And it must use the equipment and its highly trained staff in an economically efficient manner.

Consequences: Three closely related consequences of having these values, goals, and needs or purposes should be clear from the above discussion. First, the sophistication of the medical technology available and the high degree of professional care make the acute care hospital the most expensive of medical settings per patient per day. Advanced, sophisticated technologies are expensive to acquire, expensive to house and maintain, and expensive to staff. These costs must be reflected in charges for patient services.

Second, since the hospital focuses upon urgent and acute care, we come to associate the hospital with, first, the saving of life, and second, the prevention (or amelioration) of serious illness and suffering through short-term intervention (such as elective surgery or radiation therapy or chemotherapy). The general sense of the institution, therefore, is to intervene to produce marked improvement in the patient. In addition to the urgency imposed by the serious and pressing nature of the illness of the patient, the reality of high costs also fosters a sense of urgency. Patients must be treated with deliberate speed.

Third, because of high costs as well as this sense of urgency, the acute care hospital is geared toward efficiency. So that physicians may have up-to-date patient information ready at hand, progress visits are made and vital signs taken at regular intervals, even throughout the night when many patients would prefer not to be awakened. Surgical patients are aroused at 5:30 in the morning so that the surgical team can do its morning rounds before its scheduled OR time. CTscans, x-rays, and barium scans are all taken at the convenience of the diagnostic center, not of the patient. Food is served at the designated hour, not at the patient's desire. Indeed, this pressure for efficiency can produce a tendency towards authoritarianism. Allowing the patients' desires to have much play could easily lead to inefficient chaos.

12.2 The Roles of Individuals

The Physician: The hospital is the physician's "turf." The sophisticated technology, the drive towards technological intervention, and the authoritarian tendency all contribute to the marked dominance of the physician over both the patient and other members of the health care team. Indeed, the team tends to become more of a physician-ruled tool than a team of fully participatory players. With the physician in charge, care of the patient tends to be oriented towards the physician's special skills, i.e., medical intervention. The balance of power and authority subtly shifts away from the patient and members of the health care team and towards the physician.

The Patient: While the hospital is home turf for the physician, it is not for the patient. The very facts of acute and urgent illness tend to compromise their autonomy. Urgent need allows very little time to contemplate the situation in order to reach the important decisions to be made concerning treatment. Additionally, of all possible settings for health care delivery, the hospital by its very nature is the setting most alien to the patient's usual environment. The familiar landmarks of the patient's home are missing. The patient's ordinary routines have been disrupted not only by the illness itself, but also by the regimen imposed by the hospital environment.

Ethical Consequences of the Physician-Patient Roles: There are several ethical implications to be drawn from these observations. We shall discuss (1) the natural tendency of the hospital setting to diminish patient autonomy and (2) the ethical difficulties that arise when the medical care goals of the patient and the hospital are mismatched.

There are several ways in which the hospital setting tends to diminish patient autonomy. In addition to the unfamiliarity of the environment, the fact of illness tends to diminish the patient's ability to assert his autonomy. A patient confronted with an urgent and acute illness, particularly when the illness is unanticipated, is often disoriented and less able than usual to focus his or her thoughts and choose deliberately and decisively.

Furthermore, on occasion the urgency of the medical need and the consequent lack of time for thoughtful deliberation make it impossible to allow for patient autonomy. The physician's duty of beneficence becomes the guiding rule by default and decisions are made on behalf of the patient.

These factors all contribute to a tendency of the institution to dampen patient autonomy. These factors operate even in hospitals which try to promote patient autonomy. Therefore, hospitals must actively work against this institutional bias against patient self-determination.

12.3 The Hospital and Physician Autonomy

Not only is patient autonomy somewhat constrained by the hospital setting—so also is physician autonomy. This is because the hospital setting exerts pressure upon the physician to deliver care to his patients in conformity with institutional norms.

The acute care hospital is directed towards the use of sophisticated medical technology. Thus there is pressure to make use of that technology for the purpose of curing illness and saving lives, for if the technology is not being used, the question arises as to why the patient is in that hospital rather than some other care setting. The patient only has a place in the hospital when the hospital is *doing something* which other care settings cannot do. Medical residents and acute care nurses, for example, quickly get frustrated with a patient for whom they are not "doing anything."

Furthermore, since the hospital is an expensive care setting, there is strong pressure for the physician to act with deliberate speed. Changes in reimbursement schemes, such as DRGs, mean that the hospital is not compensated for the full cost of care for the patient who is being treated more slowly than necessary or not being treated at all.

Also, many hospitals are currently finding it difficult to find enough nurses to staff all their beds. As the size of the nursing staff decreases, the number of beds available for care decreases. In some cases, this has made it difficult or impossible to admit any more patients at a given time. Considerations of justice, in the sense of fairness to other potential hospital patients, require that the physician not keep a hospital bed filled with a patient who does not need and is not making use of hospital care.

Although it has been our chief concern to focus upon the similarity of values and goals among acute care institutions, one must not overlook the important fact that there are significant differences of ethical values among acute care hospitals. The most explicit case of this influence is the religious-affiliated hospital with a clearly understandable religious, ethical, and social framework which structures patient admission and care. Catholic hospitals, for example, do not allow elective abortions. More relevant to care for the elderly, the Catholic Church has been resistant to efforts to loosen the moral obligation to always provide nutrition and hydration, though the matter is one of dispute within the Catholic health care networks. Public hospitals, as a second example, have a special moral duty to provide indigent care. And teaching hospitals, as a final example, have the joint missions of providing (1) acute and urgent health care and (2) an environment conducive to quality medical education. These sorts of factors ought to be taken into account by both the health care professional and the patient in choosing between acute care institutions.

We have pointed out that acute care hospitals do have certain values, goals, and needs and purposes and that those factors can and do play an influencing role in health care delivery decisions. Though these pressures may be subtle, they can be strong. The physician will find it awkward and perhaps even unpleasant to try to care for a patient contrary to these forces. And in an important sense, it would be ethically wrong for the physician to insist upon caring for a patient in the hospital in conflict with these institutional directives, for fairness to the institution and to other patients dictates that the hospital be used according to those directives.

12.4 Hospital-Patient Mismatching

The Terms of the Mismatch: Unfortunately, cases often arise where
the values, goals and needs of patient care as understood by the
patient/family and physician are in conflict with the hospital's values, goals, and needs as an institution. This is particularly the case
with respect to care for the ill elderly, who may not share the hospital's unqualified enthusiasm for preserving life by the use of all
available medical means. The elderly eventually reach a stage in
life where death is not only the inevitable conclusion, but also a
sensible conclusion. When this stage is reached will vary greatly
from one person to another. But in some fashion or another, and at
some time or another, the concluding chapter is reached. When
the stage is reached, though one's inclination as a health care professional may be to admit the patient to the hospital, one must realize that the values and goals of the patient, as well as the goals of
medical care, may well be incompatible with those of the acute
care hospital.

The Process of Becoming Mismatched: How is it that patients
all too frequently end up "mismatched" with the acute care hospital? It tends to happen in one of two ways. The first way is through
poor planning—that is, through lack of attention or foresight on
the parts of either the health care professional or the patient/
family, the patient can be placed in an institution which is not well
matched to his or her values, goals, and needs. A very common
way in which this happens is through lack of communication between the health care professional and the patient. Not knowing
the patient's values and goals in life, the health care professional
assumes, based upon an analysis of the medical needs, that the patient must go to the hospital; whereas, given the patient's values
and goals, the hospital setting is not very appropriate. The stage is
then set for ethically troublesome conflict. The physician, feeling
the various pressures of the hospital environment, may press the
patient to accept diagnostic interventions and highly sophisticated
technological therapies which do not fit in with the patient's values and goals. The patient, perhaps feeling the pressures brought
on by dependency and the impressive authority of the physician
on his or her home turf, may wind up accepting interventions
which he or she doesn't really want just to keep the physician and
the health care team members happy. Or divisive conflict may

erupt between the patient or family and the physician and other health professionals. Careful planning, including discussion concerning values, and goals, should be employed to avoid such conflicts.

The second way in which patient-institution mismatch can arise is through unforeseeable events. A patient might be admitted to the hospital for aggressive treatment of a reversible condition, only to have a change of course in the hospital which renders the hospital treatment out of place. Yet the patient is in the hospital, and it may be awkward to transfer him or her elsewhere. This leads us back to the opening case for this chapter.

12.5 Case Revisited

The first hints of discomfort in the care of Mr. Clark came at the turn of events which prompted hospitalization. The search for reversible illnesses as an outpatient were consistent with the values and goals of care expressed by the patient and agreed to by the physician. The available diagnostic tests satisfied, at this point, the physician's need to know. However, as Mr. Clark's condition deteriorated and the evaluation was unrevealing, both felt the pressures of "need" for hospitalization.

The family appreciated the risks in the mismatch of values and goals by going to the hospital and were clear in the limitations they wished in his diagnostic and treatment plan. The patient's desires tempered his "need" for hospitalization, but it was still strong enough that he acceded to admission. The physician, on the other hand, overestimated the control he had over the environment and the success he would have in his diagnostic efforts.

The pivotal event was the patient's refusal to undergo bronchoscopy despite a lack of response to therapy and the failure of the non-invasive testing to define an etiology. It should have been concluded that the premise of the physician's "need" had been met: there was no reversible cause that he would be allowed to find. Although Mr. Clark's deteriorating condition persisted, the restrictions on interventions that he wished to maintain obviated the ability of the hospital to meet this "need." Therefore, the patient should have been discharged to his family for terminal care.

From this juncture, the story chronicals the therapeutic misadventures and withdrawal of care by the hospital staff caused by the mismatch of values, goals and needs. This became acutely obvious after the resuscitation and the failure of even the last desperate attempts at a diagnosis. It is important to note that the radiologist acted properly and in accordance with hospital policies that resuscitative efforts should be instituted first, then questions asked. The residents and nurses believed that their services were not being appropriately used, and inevitably acted on these beliefs. The physician felt trapped on the one hand by the mounting pressures of the hospital milieu and on the other by the imminence of death and a potentially litiginous family. The family sensed an estrangement from the supports they had anticipated from the staff and hospital.

Finally, although much of the responsibility rests with the physician to recognize these developments, the hospital should also provide for such circumstances. In many instances, especially in terminal illnesses, this pivotal point of mismatch is reached and there is no family to assume responsibilities. Expeditious discharge becomes impossible. With the increasing age of the hospitalized population, this situation is likely to become all too common. It is wishful thinking that in the midst of an acute care institution the staff will be able to easily accommodate these very different demands while a resolution is sought. We strongly recommend that certain areas be designated as a "step-down unit" where the values, goals and needs of the irreversibly and terminally ill may be adequately met.

12.6 Conclusion

There are two thoughts we would like to leave with the reader. First, we as members of society and as members of the health professions ought to think about what the mission of the hospital should be with respect to care for the elderly. The mission of the hospital, as understood by its administrators, physicians, and allied health professionals, has been understood as the application of sophisticated technology to cure disease and save lives. The elderly, however, are occupying an increasingly large percentage of acute care beds, and this percentage is only going to increase. Yet the elderly are persons somewhere in the last chapters of life, and death is part of that story. Hospitals could better serve this large portion of their patient population by expanding their sense of mission, not just in words but in attitudes and actions, to include care for the patient whom they cannot cure or save.

Second, physicians and other health care professionals often have a "gut feeling" that hospital care aimed at cure through intervention is out of place. Yet they may also feel pressures and inclinations to admit such patients to the hospital anyway. We have tried, in this chapter, to explain the reality behind those gut feelings. We also hope that our discussion, by clarifying the ethics at issue and how these unfortunate situations arise, may help the health care professionals and their patients in thinking through decisions concerning admission to or continuing stay in the hospital.

CHAPTER 13

The Long-Term Care Facility

The Case of "King" Pienkovitz

"King" Pienkovitz had lived at the Green Hills Nursing Center for nearly 20 years. This huge, rambling house had been converted to an extended care facility shortly after Medicare legislation was passed and had remained a favored nursing home in the heart of town. Being a bachelor and arthritic from an old injury he was no longer comfortable living alone, and so became one of the original residents. His was the turret room on the second floor, furnished with all his treasured belongings from his days as a merchant marine. He held court from his "castle" and the nurses lovingly played his maid servants—hence the epithet. Mr. Pienkovitz kept in touch with his friends from the Elks Lodge, some of whom also moved into Green Hills, forming a subsidiary men's club. They were a raucous bunch, exchanging ribald stories and playing cards in the smoke-filled day room. "King" was the perennially reelected president, presiding over club meetings with great ceremony.

The lung cancer was widespread and unresectable by the time he had developed symptoms. On his homecoming from the hospital, there was a gala celebration with a banner strung across the dayroom reading "Long Live the King" and rounds of drinking songs. But just as a party of the old guard loses something without "a little lubrication," the sight of his tired and drawn form cast a hollow ring to the joy of his return.

"King" rarely left his room. His friends in the home and from the lodge came often to spend a few hours. The nurses brought all his meals and a commode was placed next to his bed. He was always in good spirits among his friends and the staff, a man taking this turn of events with grace and self-respect. On his first post-discharge visit, he informed his physician that he had no intentions of returning to the hospital. He wished to die in his own room at the nursing home, in his own bed.

As the cancer spread, he became increasingly breathless despite the bed-side oxygen. He then developed a high fever and cough suggestive of pneumonia. The doctor ordered his transfer to the hospital. Mr. Pienkovitz refused to go. The director of nursing had the onerous duty of telling him that he could not stay. The nursing home was not equipped to manage his acute illness. They could be held responsible for not obeying the physician's orders and the home would be liable should "something bad happen." Within a few hours he was too weak to protest and an ambulance was called. He lapsed into a coma on the way and arrested in the emergency room. By the time the hospital staff learned of his underlying diagnosis and CPR status, Mr. Pienkovitz was on a respirator in the intensive care unit.

Discussion

13.1 The Long-Term Care Setting

"Long-term care" includes skilled nursing and extended care facilities, hospice care, and even domiciliary and sheltered housing. In general, long-term care is geared towards providing a protective and nurturing environment. It is a setting where patients are indeed "nursed" by their care givers. As part of an effort to convey and maintain a soothing, calm, and home-like atmosphere, urgency and commotion are discouraged.

There are several patient care goals which long-term care facilities may have. These include:

• convalescence—care designed to allow a patient the time to recover from an operation or a debilitating ill-

ness before embarking on a course of physical and oc-
cupational therapy in a milieu supportive of
functional independence before returning to the community
- skilled management of symptoms of chronic and/or irreversible illnesses—such as congestive heart failure,
chronic obstructive pulmonary disease and pressure
sores
- palliation—care designed to relieve suffering in immi-
nently terminal conditions, e.g., hospice care
- custodial care—management of chronically dependent patients, from those in coma with multiple nursing needs to a supervisory setting for those with only
cognitive incapacities.

These therapeutic goals are largely outside those of the hospital setting. Their accomplishment requires time and patience, is labor intensive and tends to be of a low technological nature.
Although efficiency in patient care management is certainly a high
priority, this is done without the exigency of acute care. There is
also an implied assurance that "everything will be taken care of"
for the comfort of the patient. The purpose of the institutions is to
provide a new home—better than that from which they came.

While there will be little or no dispute over the values and
goals noted above, there have been recent trends in long-term care
settings which tend to cloud these very values. More and more,
long-term care facilities are entering high technology care. This
has come about both because of financial incentives created by reimbursement schemes and increased professional training in the
nursing profession. Nevertheless, while taking on a more technologically sophisticated and aggressive stance, long-term care facilities have often shied away from accepting the full consequences
of providing this kind of care. After preparing the way towards
death, at least in many cases, nursing homes whisk away to an
acute care setting patients who are approaching death so that
death does not come on the premises. Promulgating the traditional goals and values of long-term care—including palliative terminal care—while providing high-tech, high-risk services, yet
succumbing to the regulations and definitions separating acute
and long-term care, has led to a kind of institutional schizophrenia. This is confusing and harmful for both the staff and the residents.

We are often uneasy about impending death, probably less so
our own than that of those close to us or under our care. This is a

natural human response. It is not surprising that long-term care residents as well as staff are not easily reconciled with death. Yet, of all health care settings, long-term care is best suited because of its mission and values to nursing the patient even as death approaches. If our patients are to receive the best of care near the end of life, that care must include the acceptance of impending death and preparation (of patient, family, and staff) for that final event.

The Physician

While the physician was clearly the dominant figure in the hospital setting, care delivered in the long-term facilities is predominantly nursing in nature. The diagnostic and therapeutic strategies which are the peculiar province of the physician are best provided in the hospital or outpatient setting. Only recently has the challenge of nursing home medicine become of growing interest in this country.

This is not to say, however, that the physician's role is unimportant. The physician traditionally has ultimate responsibility for patient care in the long-term care setting, though his role is more like that of a supervisor than a "hands-on" manager. Regulations have increasingly demanded that the physician assume responsibilities for reviewing the therapeutic plans developed by the other professional staff, establishing monitoring guidelines, recertifying needs for continued care at a specified level, and reviewing the patient's status at regular intervals. In addition, physician participation on certain quality assurance and administrative committees is mandated.

The growth of geriatric medicine has spurred interest in the complexities of long-term care as distinct from acute and ambulatory care. This development has fostered two major changes. The first has been the movement toward a higher degree of technological care, especially within skilled nursing facilities. This has included the establishment of ventilator units, capabilities for total parenteral nutrition, intensive rehabilitation, and AIDS hospices; many out-patient surgical procedures are also available within the nursing home, such as cystocopy, various endoscopies and percutaneous endoscopic gastrostomies. The second has seen a greater participation of physicians in the long-term care team. This has improved both the diagnostic and therapeutic potential within the home, but also, to some extent, the bravado in terminal care management.

If health care in the long-term care setting is to be delivered in an efficient and morally responsible manner, the physician must reach an understanding of his role within that setting, acknowledging responsibility for leadership and oversight while also acknowledging the role of the team in actual care.

The Nurse

The long-term care setting is above all the nurses' domain. While the vast bulk of patient care in the acute care hospital is actually delivered by nurses, it is delivered under the direction and close supervision of the physician. In the majority of long-term care settings, however, the physician makes only relatively rare appearances and manages the patient from afar. Thus the daily patient care responsibilities and much of the decision making fall to the nurse.

For most of its history, therefore, the long-term care setting has provided primarily custodial nursing care. In the vast majority of institutions this involves the physical care of dependent patients, including bathing, feeding, toileting and administering medications, etc. These highly personal forms of caring engender the depth of intimacy and attention which characterizes the best in long-term care.

With a greater emphasis on nursing sciences, recent graduates are better prepared for the demands of the newer technology. The shortages in nursing personnel in hospitals throughout the country have also led to more training and broader capabilities among established nurses. This knowledge has found its way into the nursing staffs of many skilled nursing facilities, as has the attraction for the technology more characteristic of the hospital.

The Administration

These recent trends have resulted in a subtle but important shift in the long-term care setting's own attitudes about its goals and mission, and an expansion of its perceived purpose. In particular, the increased use of such technology has fostered a shift towards more interventionist attitudes, in addition to the goals of palliation and custodial care, especially in the skilled nursing facilities. In addition, the enthusiasm and added capabilities of the higher level professional staff have allowed the administration to move into far more remunerative areas of care than ever before.

Several states have adopted incentive mechanisms through differential reimbursements to encourage nursing homes to take patients with greater needs and complexity of care. This trend is felt most in the extended care facilities. Custodial care now includes the management of a number of types of enteral feedings, ostomies and urinary drainage catheters. Behavioral problems, except those most severe, also come under its purview. The day is rapidly waning when many patients in nursing homes closely resemble those in domiciliary and sheltered housing.

But nursing homes are also under strict regulatory guidelines which determine types of personnel, patterns of hierarchy, and minimum numbers of nursing hours required for a specific patient. Especially in the case of Medical Assistance, the institution's standing has been tied to these minimum standards, and restrictions on the kinds of cases appropriate to an institution have also been outlined. Thus, both a "floor and ceiling" have been defined as appropriate care on a given service in a given facility. These limitations are then reflected in the care that is felt appropriate.

The Patient

Despite this small but burgeoning trend towards a more technological mode of care, most patients find the long-term care setting less alien and disorienting than the acute care hospital. It lacks the pressing urgency and the disruptive and invasive application of sophisticated and frightening diagnostic or treatment technologies. Few, however, choose to be admitted and the uncertainty, loss of privacy and control, and realization by many that this may be their last residence has a marked effect on many.

Several studies have shown that contrary to popular belief, length of stay in the nursing home is not usually long. Liu and Manton (1983) showed that approximately 60 percent of admissions within a given year have left—most alive at the time of discharge—and that only 40 percent become the "typical" patient in the nursing home. This last group lives in the home an average of two years, although the range is quite large. The period of greatest discharge rate is within the first month, then the first quarter; after six months, patients join the long-stay population (unpublished study at JIGC).

Since the length of stay for the majority of admissions is less than six months, nursing homes demands of convalescence, rehabilitation, and hospice care are quite large. Yet nursing homes are usually oriented to the long-stay patient. This is manifest in two ways. First, rehabilitation services and discharge planning are rudimentary in extended care facilities—both by regulatory restrictions and lack of the supportive milieu. Second, there is the avoidance of managing care through the terminal event in those patients who have come to die.

Thus, only for the minority of patients whose duration of stay is relatively long (usually widows over 85 years of age) does the home become a familiar surrounding. Indeed, in many of these cases, patients are allowed to bring some of their own household furnishings with them. Unfortunately, reality lurks behind the comforts of home.

13.2 The Long-Term Care Facility and Patient Autonomy

Placing an elderly patient in a long-term care facility can actually promote his or her autonomy, for in some cases the home setting has become a debilitating prison. The relief of family burdens for care can actually improve family relationships, in many cases. For some patients, either coming from the acute care hospital or coming from the home setting, the long-term care facility can be an extremely helpful environment, promoting both physical welfare and personal autonomy.

On the other hand, there are certain ethically important drawbacks to residence in the long-term care setting. These institutions, like other health care institutions, are under pressure to control costs. This means that a certain degree of efficiency is not only desirable, but economically necessary. Such efficiency often is bought by reducing the autonomy and privacy of the institution's residents. Meals are served at standard times, not necessarily when a particular resident is hungry. Likewise, bathing and other hygiene is carried out at the convenience of the staff, not necessarily that of the resident. Residents are usually forced to share a room with persons who are strangers to them. In many institutions, even a husband and wife are not accommodated together. Elderly residents who may well have recently led thriving and robust lifestyles are now restricted by the institutional needs, diminishing their sense of personal dignity.

There is also an important sense in which the resident of the long-term care facility becomes dependent upon the staff. The staff provides personal hygiene, meals, medications, etc. The inequality of this relationship between staff and resident makes it difficult to treat each other as individuals of equal moral worth. This is manifest in the frequent infantilization of the residents by staff. And it can also be a reason why residents may accept a subservient and obedient role, in essence abrogating some of their personal autonomy and dignity in exchange for attentive and kind treatment on the part of the staff.

13.4 Long-Term Care Facility and Patient Mismatching

In discussing with the elderly patient (or his or her family) the possibility of placement in a long-term care facility, the health care professional must understand that much more is at stake than the accessibility of certain types of nursing procedures or medical supervision.

First, the patient (or family) must understand both the advantages and the disadvantages of placement in a long-term care facility. What is at stake cannot be reduced to purely medical or nursing terms. Rather, the decision involves a weighing of very personal values—freedom and independence, the pleasure of living in a cherished home with pets, community, and memories—which only the patient (or when incompetent, his or her family or guardian) can make.

Second, the health care professional and the patient (or family) both must understand that the long-term care facility, just like the acute care hospital, *stands* for certain sorts of goals. Those goals, however, are significantly different from the goals of the acute care institution.

And third, the health care professional must discuss with the patient (or family) what needs the patient has which cannot be met in the home setting. Discussion is important, because the patient and professional may differ on just what those unmet needs might be.

Unfortunately, elderly patients often end up in institutions where there is little overlap in terms of values, goals, and needs. This happens in two ways. First, through poor planning the health care professional may place the elderly patient in a long-term care setting which does not match his or her values, goals, or needs. Poor planning may take a number of forms. The health care professional may operate on mistaken assumptions, perhaps even unconscious assumptions, on what the values of the patient are.

Alternatively, without the probing questioning and guidance of the health care profession, the patient may be unaware of the potential for mismatch—indeed, the patient may not have thought through the sorts of values that are at stake. The health care professional, whether the physician or a specially trained member of the health care team, must assist the patient in making this decision by helping to frame the discussion and bringing to light the important issues.

13.5 Case Revisited

The relationship between Mr. Pienkovitz and the Green Hill Nursing Center epitomizes those ethical values and goals that each wishes of the other. The patient feels a sense of comfort and belonging—of being home—and a degree of freedom to live his life within his capabilities. The home can meet his needs within their own capabilities—both in terms of service and within the confines of its governing regulations. Restrictions on alcohol and smoking become minor annoyances, accepted as facts of institutional life, but the social milieu can otherwise be recreated, which, in essence, meets his needs.

Even after the diagnosis of cancer, the home is able to meet his needs and present goals, i.e., comfort and assistance with the activities of daily living. However, there is a disquiet about the situation which comes from a shift in values on the part of Mr. Pienkovitz, not the nursing home. Green Hills is not equipped to be a hospice; their mission is to provide for a pleasant life, not a dignified death. As his symptoms progress, the nursing home becomes increasingly less supportive. The physician and nursing staff interpret his pneumonia as an acute event rather than the frequent harbinger of death and use the excuse of mismatched needs/capabilities to force his transfer to the hospital—although "anywhere else" would do.

What happens at the emergency room is totally consistent with the hospital's goals, values and purpose, which are obviously at odds with our knowledge of what Mr. Pienkovitz had wanted. Even if the diagnosis and resuscitation directives had been conveyed, the hospital staff would have been rightfully angered. But in reality, this is also far too common an occurrence for the hospital not to have been prepared.

A final important point is the home's right to transfer. Levels of care and types of services appropriate to long-term care facilities are highly regulated—as they are in hospitals. These "floor to ceiling" service boundaries are intended to assure that care is provided in a setting able to meet the patient's needs, and these regulations are enforced through reimbursement ceilings and denial of payments when a patient's needs could be met at a lower level of care. Thus, as needs change, levels of care and therefore settings of care change.

Within a strict medical model, this approach makes sense. The case of Mr. Pienkovitz, however, illustrates where this medical model fails. At the end of life, one's values and goals may significantly differ from those usually associated with a given level of need. Also, values and goals may assume a greater weight, whereas in the medical model need more often supercedes. Our current health care delivery structure has great difficulty in accommodating these differences, and therein lies the problem.

The resolution to this situation is an appreciation of these differences among the regulatory agencies and for appropriate arrangements to be made both within the acute and long-term care arenas. Of course, this is also dependent on the health care providers' ability to recognize these changes. Hospice units should be made available in both skilled nursing and extended care facilities; in other circumstances, these beds could also be used for sub-acute care. Domiciliary and sheltered housing can in large measure recreate this atmosphere through home care hospice programs. Hospitals can admit directly to their "step-down" units. And, "death with dignity" can be given a home.

13.6 Conclusion

This chapter has explored what the values, goals, and needs of the long-term care institution are and how they can match or mismatch those of the elderly patient.

We have argued that the health care professional must take a leading role in discussing with an elderly patient the possibility of placement in a long-term care facility. That discussion must cover not only the medical or nursing needs of the patient (as perceived by the health care professional) but it must also bring to light the very personal kinds of values and goals that might be promoted or threatened by moving into the long-term care facility.

We have also argued that long-term care facilities must make efforts to assist both residents and staff to understand and in a sense accept the event of death, which is the natural culmination of much of the nursing care delivered in such institutions. This is necessary if long-term care facilities are to avoid the schizophrenia which arises from holding inconsistent sets of values and goals.

References

Liu K and Manton KG. "The Characteristics and Utilization Pattern of an Admission Cohort of Nursing Home Patients," *Gerontologist* 23:92–98 (1983).

CHAPTER 14

The Home

The Case of Grandma Nell

"Grandma Nell isn't actually my grandmother, she's my father's aunt. What a character. Before she sold her car she had this bumper sticker that said, 'I hope to live long enough to be a burden to my children!' Even though she didn't have any, she sort of adopted our family and I suppose that's good enough for me.

"Well, anyway, she was living in this funky old house which she had moved into when she was only eight—that was in 1916. After she broke her hip—about five years ago—I asked her why she stayed in that huge old house. She told me that after her older sister left (that's my real grandmother) and her brother, there was nobody there to look after her parents. So, even though she got married too, she stayed to take care of her mother, who eventually died sometime in the 1940s. And then her dad died in the fifties. Gramps died about 10 years ago and now she is sort of there all by herself. But she says those ghosts keep her company and she has no intentions of leaving them behind.

"After she broke her hip, she got this boarder to live on the third floor who cooks her breakfast before she goes to work and her supper after she comes back again. Grandma Nell was doing all right, although she had to set things up on one floor because she couldn't get upstairs with her walker. A few months ago, she got sick with some middling kind of infection and her doctor put her in the hospital. Even though she was on IVs, I didn't think it was that serious, but my dad really laid it on thick. He thought she ought to go to a nursing home where they could keep an eye on her and she wouldn't have to do so much for herself. He worked out the details with her physician and she was all set to go.

"Boy, did she raise a ruckus. She fired my father. She fired the doctor. She even fired the hospital! When the ambulance crew dropped her off at her house, she warned them never to 'darken my door again!' Can't you just see it? Anyway, she's doing just fine, thank you!"

Discussion

14.1 The Home Setting

For the greatest part of its history, medicine has been practiced in the home. It was only in this century that the hospital and long-term care settings took the large role which they now have. Locating the practice of medicine in these institutions has, over the past several decades, rendered the home setting an unfamiliar locus of care for the health care professional. Yet patients, families, and third-party payors are joined in efforts to reaffirm the home as (at least in many instances) an appropriate locus for health care delivery. If we as health care professionals are to provide this care in an ethically admirable fashion, we must understand the nature of the home setting.

We do not commonly think of the home as an "institution" in the same way that we do hospitals or long-term care facilities. The home setting does indeed share many of the same characteristics in the context of health care delivery. Specifically, the home connotes certain values; it must meet certain goals for the family; and it has its own needs for maintenance of a physical and financial nature for which the family must be responsible. As in the preceding chapter, we shall clarify these values, goals and needs attributed to the home setting for long-term care, explore some important consequences of care in the community and elucidate the circumstances which may render elderly patients mismatched in this setting.

The home is a very complex, precious and diverse institution in our society. We cannot do full justice to such a central matter in only a few pages, but will focus on one pivotal theme which ties together the values, goals, and needs of the American home: independence.

Values: We can understand the home as an institution which allows a family to live relatively independent of other families. Whether a single family dwelling or an apartment, owned or leased, the home stands as a place where the family lives apart from other individuals. It is run according to the family's rules, where the family exerts its own will. It reflects the family's tastes, socioeconomic status, and often (by its location) our ethnic affiliations; it is a safe haven to which to return. And it is usually our greatest investment, our most valuable asset. Our home is very much a part of our individuality: a source of identity, the setting of our memories and a symbol of our place in society.

Goals: The home has the goals of meeting both the functional and social needs of the individuals in the family. This is very different from the hospital and long-term care facility, which reflects the needs of health care professionals and the need for cost efficient care.

The function of the home is viewed in the context of the activities of daily living. Some features stem from architectural design, for instance distances between rooms, the necessity of stairs, the widths of doorways, the placement of furnishings, and convenient access to kitchen and bathroom appliances. Although these design features are integral parts of a home they are more often chosen with the social needs in mind, i.e., the character and ambience that the home connotes. As one accrues impairments, functional convenience gains in importance, and it is here where these design features may become barriers to successful independence. Changing the home environment to facilitate functional abilities becomes as much a part of the health care plan as prescriptions and home care services.

Problems may arise when the functional needs of the patient clash with the social needs of the others in the family. The demands of care giving may significantly impair the freedoms and independence of others in the household. These mismatches between family members as to their own needs can become serious concerns.

Needs: It is also apparent that the home itself has certain needs, i.e., the home must be maintained as an independent unit. This demands two different forms of abilities from its occupants.

The first is the physical ability to clean and repair the structure. If one lives with other family members, these tasks fall to them; if alone, the extent of one's disabilities or financial resources to pay for services determines the quality of upkeep. The second is cognitive: the mental ability to get necessities (food, heat, etc.), pay bills and manage the household business. These responsibilities are obviously assumed in the hospital and nursing home, but in the community they become a major concern in developing a total health care plan.

One often overlooked concern occurs when the structure does not belong to the patient. The "needs" of the home are shared with the owner, who has a financial interest in the property. The landlord rightfully demands a certain level of maintenance and may restrict certain changes necessary in the functional support of the patient, i.e., bathroom rails, chair lifts or outdoor ramps. In apartment buildings or other congregate living situations, there will also be restrictions on behavior which may be disruptive of others. The needs of the management to provide a suitable living environment to its other tenants may supercede the freedoms of the individuals.

14.2 Consequences of the Setting

Understanding the nature of the home setting allows us to see several important ethical consequences for the delivery of long-term care services. Members of the household occasionally become ill, and family members are expected to take on the care of one another. This is quite compatible with the values and goals of the family unit and has little bearing on the home as a setting for care. However, while this may be true for illnesses of a reasonably short duration, the viability of the home, in terms of its values, goals, and needs, can be threatened by the obstacles, problems, and burdens of long-term care.

First, other members of the family must channel much of their time and energy into care of the ill person. This is no small undertaking, and one which usually entails a commitment of many years (Streib, 1972).

Second, there is the displacement of responsibilities for maintaining the home onto others in the family. These are *added* duties and, in many ways, may demand new and unfamiliar roles.

Third, there is the impingement on the social uses of the

home by others in the family. Long-term care, especially when structural changes are necessary, may change the character of the home so that it more closely resembles the hospital or long-term care facility than a private household.

And finally, the added costs of health care services and supplies not covered by most insurance programs in the community can strain the financial resources of the family.

When taken together, these pressures can create an onerous burden upon the home system in the course of extended care which can eventually threaten its continued existence as an independent place of living.

14.3 Roles in the Home Setting

The Patient: Unlike the acute care hospital or the long-term care facility, the home is the patient's "turf." The health care professional comes into the home setting by way of invitation. The patient is most likely to exercise his or her autonomy in the home setting, being more forthright about personal values because of the security and confidence supported by the familiarity of the home setting and the control exercised by the patient in that setting.

The Family: In much the same way, the family has a greater role in the home setting, both in decision making and in the health care provider's evaluations and recommendations. Several special considerations bear mentioning:

First, what care giver skills the family has must be an important factor in care delivery decisions. Do family members have the intellectual capacity to provide proper care according to sometimes complex instructions? Do they have the physical wherewithal to perform necessary care giver tasks?

Second, the health care professional must take into consideration the ability and willingness of the family to take on the financial burdens of home care. Home care services, though often less costly from an overall point of view, frequently require the patient or family to bear far more of the costs than hospitalization or care in a skilled nursing facility as follow-up to an acute illness. The financial burdens of home care could threaten the viability of the family's finances. The health care professional must consider whether the financial burden of a proposed course of home care is compatible with the financial status of the family.

Third, the family may have duties to others, e.g., other sick adults, or children, which would be compromised by home care. Does the family have a realistic view of the potential conflict of interests?

Fourth, the family can control access and therefore dictate the extent of services that may be provided. This becomes a special concern when the family may feel excessively burdened by home care demands. This creates the possibility for forms of "elder abuse." The only recourse may be through adult protective services and the courts, if the family is not cooperative.

The Physician: The patient's home is furthest from the "turf" of the physician, leading to a reversal of advantage insinuated by the settings of most other doctor-patient encounters, but one which can also provide new insights for patient care. The physician usually comes to the home alone, without the entourage of nurses and assistants who subtly support his or her viewpoint. Add to this the fact that the sophisticated technology of the acute hospital setting is less accessible, and therefore the physician must rely more fully on clinical skills, intuition and powers of persuasion in recommending diagnostic and therapeutic maneuvers. This is an alien and uncomfortable position for many physicians and, unlike other health professionals, the physician does not often choose to provide care at home but does so under the weight of the patient's circumstances. Although some might be intimidated by these disadvantages, a home visit should also be seen as an opportunity to gain valuable information not readily obtained otherwise.

First, entry into the home setting provides an opportunity for candid assessment of the patient's values and goals (as well as needs) that might not be as freely expressed or as clearly visible as in other care settings.

Second, it opens the possibility for an assessment of the family's status and their ability and willingness to support the patient's health care needs. The home setting can help the family to share their concerns and to demonstrate their commitment to the care of the patient in a way that is not feasible in other settings. The health care professional sensitive to the dynamics of the home setting assumes a role far more that of counselor and advisor than the dictatorial promulgator of the health care plan. Third, there is an opportunity for educating the family in the skills necessary for the care of the patient. This can only be done in the abstract in the office or in the hospital, but in the home this training takes on very concrete terms.

Team Members: On several occasions, it has been pointed out how the team approach to health care is of particular value for the elderly. Nurses, therapists, and social workers all play a crucial role in helping the elderly person maintain that functional independence which is necessary for well-being in the community. This is especially true in the context of home care. Yet, because of a lack of a central location, the practice of team care poses several ethical issues.

First, in delivering home care and in making care decisions and recommendations, team members have relatively more importance and responsibility than they do in the hospital setting. This is partly because the home is not the physician's turf. It is also partly because team members are likely to have contact with the patient which is more frequent and of a longer duration than physician-patient contact. This entails greater authority as well as greater moral responsibility for team members.

Second, the lack of a centralized locus of care can make it difficult to coordinate care planning and care activity among the various team members. It is essential for effective care that each member fosters coordination and cooperation within the team.

Third, each member must assume responsibilities for alerting others on the team to needs outside their own expertise. This requires a broadening of one's professional perspective beyond the usual scope of services and accepting an obligation to assume certain case management functions which may not have been included in one's own training. This is especially true considering (a) the significant possibilities of non-adherence and non-compliance and (b) the increasing presence of technology in the home which may be used in a mistaken and harmful manner.

Fourth, each member must accept responsibility for bringing lapses in the quality of care to the attention of the team. This can be a particularly unwelcome and unappealing duty. Yet while poor care may be relatively obvious when seen in the acute or long-term care facility, it is not public when it occurs in the home setting. The duty to stand forward and report it, therefore, becomes proportionately stronger.

14.4 Home-Patient Mismatch

The Mismatch: As has been pointed out in preceding chapters, it is advantageous to all involved that the values, goals, and needs of the patient correspond to those of the care setting. It is ethically important to try to avoid patient-setting mismatches. Let us consider three ways in which an elderly patient can become mismatched with his or her own home.

The first mismatch is along functional parameters. The layout of the rooms and the architectural barriers of stairs, doorways or inaccessible kitchen and bathroom appliances may render the environs unsuitable. If he or she is unable to stock adequate food stores, or is unable to prepare proper meals, or even use the bathing and toileting facilities, that patient's health is threatened. Where the patient is not the owner, restriction on structural changes may severely limit the adaptation of the home to meet their needs.

The second mismatch arises when the patient is no longer able to carry out the activities necessary for the continuance of the home as a setting of care. This is particularly the case when the person in question does not live with any responsible adult spouse, friend or offspring. If disability precludes basic home cleaning and maintenance, the structural integrity and safety of the home is jeopardized. Should the patient no longer be able to keep home finances straight, and bills are not paid, essential utilities could be lost. Broadly understood, then, a person's inability to fulfill the physical and cognitive demands of the home puts the feasibility of home care into question since it puts the independence of the home at risk.

The third mismatch is when the needs of the patient place burdens upon the family which the family cannot or will not accept. When a family member requires extensive home care, the burdens of both patient care and household management often fall to other adult family members either in the home or nearby. Although most families are willing to pick up these responsibilities for some time, extended demand upon them as care givers draws their time and resources away from other duties and is a source of increasing stress. Especially when this is an unexpected and unwanted role, the frustration, resentment, and sheer exhaustion can turn what had been constructive and helpful relationships into those which are resentful and destructive. Neither the family nor the patient is benefited by such a situation.

Avoiding Mismatches: The first step in avoiding patient-home mismatches is to base home care and/or discharge planning and recommendations upon accurate assessments of the patient's values, goals, and needs in relation to those of the home and responsible family members. This assessment includes both an objective assessment of the patient's medical, nursing, and social needs and an understanding of the family's values and goals in relation to those needs.

We have found that a viable approach is to perform our functional assessments in the context of a "Patient-Caregiver Unit." This is a two-part evaluation instrument (currently under development and testing) which measures both the functional abilities of the patient and the care giver, as well as their motivation to maintain community independence. Where the patient demonstrates an area of dependency, the primary care giver is assessed in both the ability and willingness to assume responsibility. If both are lacking, we assess the availability (and affordability) of formal care giver services through agencies and volunteer organizations. This provides a more realistic appraisal of the potential success of long-term care in the community.

Assessment of the nursing and social needs can best be done by a home visit which allows a functional evaluation within the context of the actual living environment. An understanding of the patient's values and goals in developing a mutually acceptable treatment plan is best achieved by frank and extended conversation with the patient (and his or her family). As already argued, the home setting can actually be most conducive to such a discussion. The patient is on his or her own territory and not confused or intimidated by the alien environment of the acute care hospital.

On the other hand, when the home environment is clearly seen as a great risk, the characteristics of the setting put the health care provider at a substantial disadvantage in negotiating an alternative. The very fact that the patient is home may lead to a certain bravura—and inappropriate decisions may be made. It is sometimes necessary to change the setting of the negotiations, even under court order, so as to bring the concerns to light.

14.5 Moving the Patient from the Home Setting

Moving is generally prompted by an increasing discordance between the goals of the patient and the family or the ability to meet the physical and financial needs required for maintenance of the structure. However, in any move, it is important to appreciate that the values of the home ought to be transferred as well.

The goals of privacy and independence may become superceded by the needs of the individual for care and a supportive environment. Physical barriers within the home may preclude access to essentials, distance from family may make care unfeasible, or the expense of restructuring the home and purchasing services may be beyond the family's means. The second reason for considering a change of residence is when the maintenance needs of the structure exceed either the physical or economic abilities of the family. This is most often the situation when an older couple or parent are left alone in the family home and failing health obviates their ability to manage. In both these instances, the conflicts of needs loom larger than the hold of memories, traditions and other family values.

When the competent individual elects to move late in life, it is usually prompted by a rational wish to choose a new setting in better accord with his or her current or anticipated needs. Problems may arise when "family values" held by others intercedes in this decision. There may be a wish to maintain the home as a "monument," or as an expected inheritance. Although these issues add to the emotional burdens of moving, they should be identified as extraneous to the more basic motivations for this choice.

The more difficult circumstance is when the individual is marginally or fully incompetent and therefore unaware of the discordance created by his or her illness. Family or social agencies are then given the onerous responsibility of effecting the move. A general rule to follow would be that the patient should participate in the selection of the new residence and processes of moving in direct proportion to their awareness of the problems. For the willing but incompetent, the patient should be told of the intentions to stay elsewhere and that remembrances from home should be brought to the new location. For the recalcitrant, incompetent patient it may be necessary to engage the assistance of adult protective services, or perhaps the courts. Efforts should be made to ease the transition. Sedation should be avoided if at all possible, and the family should be strongly encouraged to visit frequently during the transition.

14.6 Death in the Home Setting

Given the evolving values, goals and needs of formal health care settings, it is again falling to the home to become the preferred place of death. Our society and our profession became so enamored of the burgeoning technology and abilities to delay dying over these past few decades that death more frequently came in the midst of continued therapeutic attempts in the hospital. Sometimes the paternal wish to protect families from the fears, discomforts and unsightliness of death encouraged us to institutionalize this event. As we have also grown to accept our limitations and to question the wisdom of futile efforts at the end of life, we have also grown to appreciate that death is predominantly a family affair and should take place in the family setting whenever possible.

Unfortunately, few young people have experienced a planned death at home and the customs which provided family support have waned. It becomes our responsibility as primary care providers to reintroduce this practice, despite the personal burdens it may entail, and to encourage our patients and their families to seriously consider this option. We hope that the principles and skills expounded in this book will facilitate the task. The results may be a better appreciation of the issues of the health care setting, and help in easing the ethical burdens of medical management at this time in life.

14.7 Case Revisited

Grandma Nell had been able to change her environs and develop a "family" to supplement for her disabilities. She met the requirements of providing for both her own and her home's needs. The care giving responsibilities were acceptable to the boarder and allowed her the freedoms of a job and social life within her own quarters. Grandma Nell's relatives only had to provide moral support and a degree of supervision. The sense of satisfaction in the case stems from the fact that Grandma Nell could overcome a challenge to this arrangement and maintain her independence.

Once hospitalized, the picture of a recently ill, walker-dependent elderly woman living alone in a large house with many stairs would suggest a substantial risk on discharge. The doctor and the nephew saw Grandma Nell out of context, extrapolating her needs in the hospital to her home and concluding that she would be unsafe at home. In the hospital, they felt on firm ground in making these plans on her behalf, and it was only through sheer dint of her will that they did not succeed. Yet these same needs, when seen in the context of her molded environment, would have led to a totally different viewpoint.

This case illustrates a phenomenon common to those who limit their work predominantly to hospitals and their private office. It takes many years to gain an appreciation or knowledge of the lifestyles, family and community support systems, and the determination to maintain independence against incredible odds that characterize our patients. Residents in training often see people as if they arrived at the hospital or offices from some black hole only to return when we are through with our ministrations. This viewpoint is obviously very limiting in making decisions concerning discharge planning. But the opportunities for developing this awareness must be sought through experience and taught by example in order to accord the professional prestige in providing care at home its proper perspective.

14.8 Conclusion

The home as a distinct setting of care with its own ethical value system is not often considered, yet it has been estimated that there are from one to three patients cared for in the community for every patient in a nursing home (National Nursing Home Survey, 1977). This would make the home the largest setting for health care delivery. This population is likely to grow as our society ages, as regulations are enacted to reduce hospital lengths of stay, and as the number of nursing home beds remain limited by government restrictions.

Unfortunately, our professional training and experience are too often limited in the knowledge and skills of effective management of patients in their own environments, or in assessing the home as an appropriate place for care. By acquiring a broader understanding not only of the values, goals and needs imbued in the home, but also the abilities of the family and the community to provide the necessary social supports and health care services, we may make better decisions in planning for the long-term care of our patients and assuring their long-term well-being.

Permutations

A most significant change in this story would be if Grandma Nell had not owned her home. This presents the issue of shared autonomy in which both the patient and the property owner would have to agree on her returning home. Although a landlord's decision not to allow a tenant to return home for reasons of ill health would be subject to regulations governing evictions, this decision would override the wishes of the patient if it could be shown that the needs of the property were in jeopardy.

References

Streib G. "Older Families and Their Troubles: Familial and Social Responses," *Family Coordinator* 21:5–19 (1972).

Part IV

The Impact of Reimbursement Policies on Medical Decision Making

CHAPTER 15

Ethics, Reimbursement and Decision Making

The Case of Mr. Leopold

Mr. Leopold was already an old man at 68. He had been an artist before the stroke three years ago left him paralyzed on his right side and aphasic. Although the artistic side of his brain was not affected, he was unable to translate his thoughts into comprehensible, let alone sellable paintings. And, of course, he could no longer teach.

A man of intellect, sensitivity and passion, as well as a pragmatist, he married into a relatively wealthy family. Income from a trust established by Mrs. Leopold's parents, supplemented by his teaching and the occasional sale of paintings from his gallery, supported the family modestly but comfortably. Their trust income was substantially reduced by the inflation of the 1960s and 1970s, but Mr. Leopold was becoming more established during this period, so that the losses were not fully appreciated. Until the stroke.

Mrs. Leopold was able to maintain the gallery through commissions from the sale of paintings and sculptures by Mr. Leopold's former students. The law firm on the first floor that owned the building in which they had their gallery and apartment was very understanding, and relaxed the rent obligations. In time, the turmoil of these events subsided and Mr. and Mrs. Leopold settled onto a stable, though lower, economic rung.

Last year, Mrs. Leopold sold her parents' home, which she had inherited, to help their only child buy a house in California.

This past Christmas Eve, Mr. Leopold developed an acute abdomen requiring surgery to remove his gangrenous gallbladder, followed by a urinary tract infection with sepsis. These back-to-back insults rendered him weak, totally dependent and demoralized. Mrs. Leopold felt that she would be unable to manage him at home, and the discharge plans seemed to point towards nursing home placement.

Mrs. Leopold soon discovered that her husband was not eligible for medical assistance, not because of his income—that was certainly low enough—but because of the income from the recently sold property! The dispersing of assets to his family at a time when he was already disabled was considered a purposeful divestiture. They would have to pay the state the equivalent amount of these monies in order to meet the spend-down criteria! Medicare would no longer support his hospital stay, and at an intermediate level of care, he was also not eligible for temporary institutional support. Their daughter could possibly contribute a few thousand dollars, but without assurances of continued payments, the nursing homes Mrs. Leopold contacted were not inclined to take the chance of accepting him.

And so Mr. Leopold returned home.

Discussion

There are several reasons why a discussion of the finances of health care for the elderly is particularly pertinent to a study of ethics and health care for the elderly. As a frequent consequence of aging and disease, the elderly are subject to a variety of physical and functional impairments, and therefore increased needs for health care services. This is reflected in their consumption of far more health care resources per capita than any other age group. Placed in the context of the demographic shifts in our society, the challenge of financing care for the aged has become a growing concern for both the individual and the government. Health care professionals play a pivotal role in driving the costs of care. Attention to the economic impact of our decisions will undoubtedly become a major determining factor in choosing diagnostic and therapeutic interventions, as well as in making recommendations for settings of care.

The broadest effort to address the problems of providing for the aged came when Congress enacted Medicare and Medicaid legislation in 1965 in affirmation of the belief that all older persons should have access to high quality health care without regard to their own financial resources. The initial focus of these programs, however, was on assuring the availability of acute care services, predominantly throughout the not-for-profit and government sectors. The development of long-term care services largely fell to private investors who fostered the growth of the nursing home industry with profit-making intentions. The bulk of responsibility for quality assurance and funding of long-term care for those who could no longer pay was subsumed under the state Medicaid programs.

These programs have been both blessing and bane. Government sponsorship assured payment for services and spurred the growth and utilization of hospitals and nursing homes. Hospitals and practitioners were given a virtual carte blanche and health care expenditures escalated, fueled by the expansion of medical technology which evolved from the dramatic advances in scientific knowledge over the past several decades. The effects on the long-term care industry were also impressive. The numbers of nursing home beds surpassed those in hospitals; the potential patient population seemed infinite. However, while acute care was largely subsidized by Medicare, funding for long-term care through Medicaid was not made available until the patient became impoverished.

The combination of demographics and the mounting costs of these advances in medical science and technology have, however, made the long-term survival of such programs highly tenuous in their present form. An ever greater percentage of our nation's gross national product is being spent on health related services. Medicare expenditures have risen at an average rate of approximately 7 percent per patient per year which, because of the aging of our society, represents an average increase of 18 percent in the Medicare budget each year since 1970. As Daniel Callahan has argued (1987), we cannot afford to carry this huge burden without spending less in other areas. The picture is even more problematic when one notes that almost three-quarters of Medicaid expenditures, a program originally created to provide access to health care for the poor in general, are now devoted to the care of the elderly, mostly for long-term care services in nursing homes which are not covered by Medicare.

In response to this burgeoning financial pressure on the economy, the government has instituted cost control measures and limited the extent of covered services. The elderly now pay approximately 25 percent of their health care costs from personal funds. Although this represents only 3 percent of hospital and 26 percent of physician costs, the expenditures for long-term care are 50 percent and nearly 60 percent for other health care services. Nor have private health insurers disdained such cost-control mechanisms. Thus, the health care provider for the elderly operates in a context of increasing third-party payor oversight and restriction and greater out-of-pocket remuneration from elderly patients.

Another approach to stemming the government's financial burdens for health care has been to encourage the development of prepaid arrangements through health maintenance organizations (HMOs) and other managed care options. This tactic shifts the responsibilities for cost containment onto the provider while limiting the government's liability. Although the early experiences seemed quite favorable, the profitability of these programs was eventually found to depend on their ability to attract healthy older adults. As this initial population aged, however, the profit margin diminished substantially, leading some HMOs to either further withhold services or face bankruptcy.

Nonetheless, there continues to be an emphasis on this approach. The latest development in this area is the social health maintenance organization, a demonstration project under the auspices of the Health Care Financing Administration, which targets a more representative elderly population of patients and offers a broader spectrum of services. Also in the initial planning stages is the Medicare Insured Group, a capitated health care package administered through pension plans for retirees of contracting companies and unions. Regardless of the eventual organizational structure, the commitment to pre-paid services for the elderly is clear and would appear to be enduring.

In the acute care arena, government efforts in prospective

payment have taken the form of diagnosis related groups (DRGs), a mechanism of bunching similar illnesses requiring similar resources and reimbursing the hospital a set amount for each grouped diagnoses based on an average cost per patient per admission. Provisions are made for advanced age and, to a limited extent, the complexity (but not the severity) of illness. Hospitals profit by providing services for less than the set sum, and lose money if the actual cost is more than that allotted. In effect, this places the hospital at financial risk (rather than Medicare or Medicaid) and puts the physician in the middle, balancing the patient's needs and the utilization of hospital services.

Whatever one's beliefs concerning the justice or injustice of current funding mechanisms, the practicing health care professional must accept that these systems are in place and that we must work within this framework. Financial considerations, including reimbursement sources and policies, are unavoidably a part of the framework of the provider-patient relationship and must be acknowledged and incorporated into the clinical decision-making process. It is clearly becoming the responsibility of the health care professional to assure that services are provided within the patient's means. While it is beyond the scope of this chapter to discuss specific health care policies and what constitutes a morally justifiable financing system, we will attempt to develop a framework which helps to identify the ethical complexities of these policy and financial considerations in the care of the elderly.

15.1 Types of Reimbursement Arrangements

For the purposes of this discussion, we have devised a scheme that identifies the three general types of reimbursement and three types of financially motivated conflicts concerning treatment choices. Let us begin by identifying the different types of financial arrangements.

> I.   Personally financed: All costs of care are borne by individuals from their own resources. We have purposefully excluded any outside public or private funds from this category to better illustrate the ethical issues.
>
> II. Third party based fee-for-service: A significant por-

tion of the health care costs are borne by the patient's insurance program so that the deductibles and co-payments are no longer considered deterrents to seeking care.

III. Capitation of prepaid programs: Funds for health care are paid prospectively into a group account from which the organization derives both its working capital and money for providing care of the enrollees. The organization, therefore, determines the types and extent of services offered, and the eligibility criteria for joining.

15.2 Types of Ethical Conflicts Arising from Payment Mechanisms

Our discussion will build upon three different types of financially mediated conflicts concerning treatment options.

A. *Patient-Provider Conflict Where Patient Wants Less:* By this we mean disagreement between the patient and the provider concerning how the patient's money should be spent for health care. It must be assumed that all parties are operating under the rules of professional integrity.

In these matters, the health care professional, because of his or her special training and expertise, naturally takes on the role of advisor concerning the possible options for care. It is the physician's responsibility to clarify the relative importance and value of a specific diagnostic and therapeutic approach for the patient's consideration. Financial constraints must be balanced by the weight of necessity in these negotiations.

However, health care is not usually the patient's only concern. Other financial priorities may lead the patient to prefer less testing or treatment than the health care professional might wish. Given the nature of existing reimbursement systems, particularly for long-term care and home care, "the best care medically possible" can easily lead to financial ruin for the family. The patient's decision to refrain from expensive treatment, when based upon competent and informed choice, deserves respect.

B. *Patient-Provider Agreement But Insufficient Financial Resources:* In this instance, the patient and provider are in agreement concerning what sort of treatment would be desirable, but sufficient funding for that treatment is not available.

Although Medicare covers many services, it is not all-encompassing. For example, the health care professional and the patient might agree that residence at home with home health care (which the patient cannot afford out-of-pocket) would be the best alternative. But in many localities such care would not be covered through either Medicare of Medicaid, and the patient would seem not to have access to that health care option.

C. *Patient-Provider Conflict Where Patient Wants More Than Provider Thinks Appropriate:* The physician has certain obligations to assure the appropriate use of health care services. As noted in chapter 8, there is no obligation to provide care that is medically useless. One reason, of course, is that it could be harmful to the patient. Another, however, and the one which concerns us here, is that such treatment is a waste of valuable and perhaps scarce resources.

15.3 An Analytical Matrix

Figure 2 shows the matrix of the various combinations of these ethically important factors:

Figure 2

	A Patient Wants Less Than Provider	B Patient and Provider Agree But No Funds	C Patient Wants More Than Provider
I. Paid From Personal funds	A-I	B-I	C-I
II. 3rd Party Fee-For-Service	A-II	B-II	C-II
III. Prepaid or Capitation	A-III	B-III	C-III

A-I and A-II: In both A-I and A-II sufficient funds are available for treatment which the health care professional thinks appropriate. It is just that the competent patient would prefer not to use resources for that treatment or care. This is particularly understandable when it is the patient's own resources (or the resources of the family) which are threatened. It may be more valuable to the patient to live financially independent from his or her offspring than to receive the treatment in question. Less likely, though still possible, is that case of the very altruistic patient who would prefer that society not pick up such an exorbitant bill for health care which is only slightly beneficial.

In the case of patient decision to refrain from care of treatment options because of expense, the health care provider must recognize the moral right of the patient to make these determinations. If the provider feels that to continue to care for such a patient would be to compromise his or her sense of professional integrity, the professional has a right to withdraw from the case if doing so would not constitute abandonment.

A-III: This case is similar to A-I and A-II in that the patient refuses to comply with the recommendations of the health care group. In this instance, there arises a sense of moral fairness to the physician's organization which might make for a stronger obligation to transfer care to another provider group. This is especially true in cases where choosing to forego certain kinds of standard care or treatment could foreseeably lead to a need for much more expensive care in the near future. To accommodate such a patient's wishes could place an untoward burden upon other patients within the provider group or limit resource availability in the future for more justifiable care.

B-I: A most uncomfortable circumstance arises when the physician and the patient agree on a treatment plan but the patient cannot afford the diagnostic tests or medications. We as a society have mandated that acute care be available to everyone through the public system, but our society has not chosen to make basic or primary health care a right for members of our society. Private health insurance often fails to cover all contingencies—around 36 million Americans do not have health insurance.

In the B-I type of case we might appeal to a sense of charity on the part of health care institutions and individual providers. We definitely have a moral obligation to provide a reasonable amount of *pro bono* care on an individually determined, voluntary basis. But in the end, the health care professional does not have the right or the legal ability to force health care providers to be charitable.

There are limits to the amount of philanthropy that an institution or private practitioner can carry without unfairly risking financial insolvency.

The answer must be that until we have different social policies, the lack of funds means that care—especially very expensive care—may be denied.

B-II and B-III: B-II and B-III add the factor of spending the monies of a third party into the clinical negotiations between patient and physician. The health care professional is placed in the role of gatekeeper, arbitrating the balance between the needs of the patient and the desires for efficient and cost-effective spending of assets by the insuring organization. There are subtle but important differences, however. In B-II, the patient and physician have the right to fully exercise their decisions within certain larger boundaries as defined by regulations, while in B-III the effort is to provide only that which is clearly needed and to minimize expenses through tight cost-efficiency measures.

In B-III, the health care professional and the patient are operating within a closed system, i.e., savings made in one area will be available for use in other areas within the same system. On the other hand, if the physician were to manipulate the system to get expensive care for an individual patient, there is the danger of impoverishing the organization to the detriment of other patients (Cassel 1985). The health care professional has a moral obligation to balance the relative value of a treatment plan for an individual with the needs of the population covered by the organization. The moral basis for withholding expensive care under B-III is that one is obliged to provide the best health care possible (a) to the group *as a whole* and (b) within the financial limits which constitute the group.

Several points should be kept in mind. First, patients have accepted these constraints by joining a closed financial system. The savings sought in the costs of their personal health care are based on an expectation of efficient service, closely scrutinized spending and limitations on availability and access which applies to all members, including themselves. Second, the health care professional has elected to work within these constraints as well. There remains a moral obligation to advocate on behalf of one's patient before the system, and the system should certainly be willing to consider such requests, but the patient and the provider must understand the potential for being excluded from certain options for the benefit of the organization. Third, we find it ethically unacceptable to withhold medically indicated care in a capitation or pre-paid system when doing so is motivated by any special financial bonus to the health care professional as an individual.

The response to restrictions of covered services under B-II is somewhat less clear, since savings in one instance will not necessarily assure additional funds for the health needs of others. The bounds of the allocated resources are not as explicit. According to Cassel (1985), this implies that one's moral obligations for conservation are not quite as strict as within a closed system. The proof of value to the individual of a diagnostic or therapeutic intervention need not be as definitive; patients' desires or convenience may be more readily considered in decision making. This means that one is free to accept a stronger advocacy role for the patient, negotiating with the third party for more extensive coverage to the full limits of eligibility.

C-I: This category addresses those cases where the patient wants more care than the physician thinks is medically necessary, but the individual patient (or family) is willing to pay for that care so that others are not financially penalized. In many instances it would be ethically permissible for the health care professional to provide such services, as long as there is no deleterious effect on other patients or potential harm to the individual. One should not cooperate in providing these relatively unnecessary services when they entail the use of scarce space or equipment which might be required for the care of patients who truly need those services, for example, intensive care unit beds, CAT scans, transfusions, etc. Nor should the requested diagnostic test or therapy be made available if doing so entails a substantial risk. This may represent either potential harm to the individual, e.g., medication side effects or interactions, or added risks to the community, as in the case of indiscriminant antibiotic use which may promote the emergence of resistant strains of bacteria.

C-II and C-III: In these cases, the health care professional must be willing to accept the role of gatekeeper, protecting the assets of the insurers of care. In both of these circumstances, allowing the patient to receive costly but unnecessary care unjustly affects the finances and health care of other patients. Unnecessary use of services reimbursed by third parties can translate directly into 1) higher health care costs for the government and for taxpayers, 2) higher individual insurance premiums, 3) fewer available health care services to all other members of closed health care systems. The practitioner should attempt to educate the patient as to the reasoning behind this decision, but ultimately it is the professional's moral duty in such circumstances to deny testing or treatment.

15.3 The Health Care Professional's Role in Advance Planning

The fact that finances play such an influential role in medical ethics in the care of the elderly make these considerations a topic which requires attention and guidance from the patient prior to and throughout the course of treatment. Just as we strongly advocate advance directives for defining the parameters of intervention, we strongly encourage physicians to take a more active role in assisting patients with their financial affairs. There are three issues which the health care professional should discuss: 1) the realities of insurance coverage; 2) a limited but candid discussion of the patient's wishes in disbursement of his or her estate; and, 3) funeral planning. While not specifically ethical issues, these all entail decisions which will bear upon more identifiable concerns that arise with advancing disability and eventual death.

Financial realities: According to a recent national survey by AARP, 79 percent of the people at large and 70 percent of those over 65 believed that Medicare would cover a prolonged nursing home stay. Half those with Medicare and a Medi-Gap policy thought they were fully covered for long-term care services. The lifetime risk of institutionalization is 20 percent and appropriate planning for this eventuality can be very important. Given this widespread misunderstanding of the economic realities of health care (particularly chronic care and the potential economic drain upon the patient and family) the health care professional has a moral responsibility to make an effort to educate the elderly patient and his or her family in this aspect of care. Other issues worthy of discussion might include such matters as Life-Care, long-term care insurance, and the possibility of timely disbursement to qualify for Medicaid without being required to spend all the family's wealth.

Estate planning: The second issue of wills and estate planning is one rarely addressed by physicians, but one which deserves attention. We suggest there is a professional responsibility to broach these matters when appropriate, e.g., in the care of the terminally ill. Such recommendations may help to guide the patient and family in beginning the process and in understanding the obligations and family priorities in shaping future decisions. We have found this an excellent opportunity for reassessing with the patient such options as the Living Will or durable power of attorney for health matters. The family discussions which ensue greatly clarify advance directives and immeasurably facilitate care at the end of life.

Funeral planning: The third issue is funeral planning. Physicians have a unique opportunity to address financial planning of the funeral since they are frequently aware of the impending death and are looked to for prognostic judgments. Discussing the concepts—not really the details—offers another opportunity to enhance and encourage patient autonomy. It brings the imperative to settle one's estate into sharper focus, and therefore helps in resolving many other intra-family issues. Contrary to being perceived as morbid or defeatist, our experience has been very favorable in the right situation. Patients who are aware of their terminal state and have grown to a point of acceptance or have voiced their preference for death are very likely to receive this discussion well. It also provides the opportunity to readdress the issues of the durable power of attorney or Living Will at a time when this information takes on greater urgency.

These topics should be raised in private with the patient or, if incompetent, with the person designated as the decision maker. If the patient so desires, the family may be brought into the discussion at an early stage. Once decisions are reached, a more public discussion often helps families appreciate the gravity of the illness. This then allows time for rational and deliberate planning and to prepare for mourning.

15.4 Case Revisited

The dilemmas of Mr. and Mrs. Leopold illustrate two sides of the same problem. Theirs is not really a study of government intrusion forcing an unfavorable health care option, but rather a study in difficult choices in which money plays a central role.

From the perspective of the patient and his family, the Leopold's had to choose between supporting their daughter in her new home or reserving this money for easily foreseeable health care needs. Once this decision was made, they were obligated to deal with its consequences. In truth, there were other options which they did not care to pursue, such as moving to California with their daughter, separation and divorce (which technically would leave Mr. Leopold without means of support), or living with another relative or friend willing to accept their income in exchange for room, board and compensation for secondary care giver assistance. In fact, Mrs. Leopold was able to take her husband home with the aid of the home care program and additional durable medical equipment. There they are managing, although with some difficulty.

Two issues should be addressed from the government's perspective. The first is that it was the presence of Medicaid as a source of funding which raised the possibility of institutional placement on discharge from the hospital. This fact raises the likelihood that demand for nursing home services will increase as a result of the increasing prevalence of long-term care insurance. This would substantially change the financing of institutionalization from one which is personally funded to a third-party mechanism of funding, with secondary implications in changing the locus of control. Placement decisions will undoubtedly involve many more considerations as private insurers enter this market in the near future.

The second issue is that the government must protect itself from purposeful distribution of assets by the patient or the family. Since Medicaid assumes responsibility for financial support, it reserves the right to determine the guidelines under which support is offered, i.e., after depletion of all but a minimum of private resources ("spend-down"). It is important to appreciate this fiduciary right. Irretrievably investing in non-health-related expenditures would become a means for the family to divert its financial resources for personal gain while the government, through general tax revenues, must support the health care needs of the individual. Clearly it is unfair to hold the public responsible for paying for health care which the family has found a low priority. As "emissaries of health," physicians should alert their patients to this reality.

15.5 Conclusion

Health care professionals have frequently espoused the view that they should make care decisions without regard to financial considerations, that their concern should be only the welfare of the patient, not the pocketbook. On the contrary, such deliberate refusal to confront and deal with the economic realities of health care can be an unethical disservice to the individual, the family, and the larger community. The morally responsible health care professional should be sensitive to the conditions under which financial considerations ought to be given ethical weight in making treatment and care decisions for an individual patient. The point of this chapter has been to provide an analytical framework for clarifying the possible situations in which financial concerns may arise, and what would (in our opinion) be the ethical approach to take in these different circumstances.

As practicing health care professionals, we may be unhappy with the manner in which various reimbursement systems are structured. In particular, we may dislike existing governmental policies restricting the access of our elderly patients to appropriate health care options. Governmental policies concerning long-term care and home care in particular pose troubling ethical questions. It is certainly a duty of the health care professional to play a leading role in public debate concerning national, state, and local health care policies.

Annotated Bibliography

American College of Physicians. "Financing Long-Term Care," *Annals of Internal Medicine* 108: 279–88 (1988).
  This article by the Health and Public Policy Committee of the ACP reviews current methods of financing long-term care and problems with current policies. It puts forward several suggestions on alternative financing mechanisms, analyzing the advantages and disadvantages of various proposed schemes.
Bayer R and Callahan D. "Medicare Reform: Social and Ethical Perspectives," *Journal of Health Politics, Policy and Law,* 10: 533–47 (1985).
  Bayer and Callahan trace Medicare from its origins to its present state, arguing that the ethical rationale for its creation may no longer apply in light of other growing and unmet health care needs.

Cassel CK. "Doctors and Allocation Decisions: A New Role in the New Medicare," *Journal of Health Politics, Policy and Law,* 10: 549–64 (1985).
Physicians increasingly are being asked to play a role in conserving economic resources by curbing use of health care. Cassel argues that this would be acceptable morally only if (1) there is universal access to basic care, (2) physician income is not directly related to treatment choices, (3) savings from restricting use stay within the health care system, and (4) an ethically acceptable decision procedure exists for allocation decisions.

Feinstein RJ. "Physician Payment Plans and Conflicts of Interest," *Journal of the Florida Medical Association,* 73:387–89 (1986).
Feinstein points out that it has become increasingly common to offer financial inducements to physicians in pre-paid plans to keep costs low. While not attacking the concept of pre-paid plans in general, Feinstein does argue that they should be structured so that such financial conflicts of interest between the patient's care and the physician's financial remuneration are minimized.

References

American Association of Retired Persons. *Long Term Care Research Study,* Washington, D.C.: AARP, 1984.
Cassel CK. "Doctors and Allocation Decisions: A New Role in the New Medicare," *Journal of Health Politics, Policy and Law,* 10:549–64 (1985).
Committee on Nursing Home Regulation, Institute of Medicine. *Improving the Quality of Care in Nursing Homes,* Washington, D.C.: National Academy Press, 1986.
Keeler EB, Kand RL, Solomon DH. "Short and long-stay residence of nursing homes." *Med Care* 19:363–70 (1981).
United States Special Committee on Aging, American Association of Retired Persons, The Federal Council on Aging and the Administration on Aging. *Aging America: Trends and Projections, 1985–86,* Washington, D.C.: Department of Health and Human Services, 1986. (Publication no. 498-116-814/42395).
Vladek BC. *Unloving Care: The Nursing Home Tragedy,* New York: Basic Books, 1980.
Vogel RJ, Palmer HC. *Long-Term Care: Perspectives From Research and Demonstrations,* Rockville, MD: Aspen Publications, 1985.

Glossary of Ethical Terms

The brief glossary below is a short list of the ethical terms with which the reader should be familiar. For the reader who wishes to pursue ethical theory more generally, there is a short bibliography of educational texts in medical ethics listed at the end of the glossary.

AUTONOMY—

Autonomy literally means "self rule." It refers to a person's capacity to make reasoned choices concerning what he or she will do and how he or she will be treated.

Our society now generally agrees that the health care professional has a moral obligation to respect the autonomy of the patient. This belief is reflected in the legal emphasis upon one's obligation to obtain *informed consent* from patients before engaging in any significant medical or diagnostic intervention.

Numerous arguments have been given as to why we have a moral obligation to respect each other's autonomy. Immanuel Kant argues that it is the possession of rational will that makes us moral agents. Thus, to treat another person as though he or she did not have a rational will is to denigrate his or her status as a person. John Stuart Mill, on the other hand, argued that to frustrate or override another person's ability to make personal choices seriously harms that individual. Disregarding the rights of other persons to make their own choices unnecessarily constricts the freedom of the other person and creates a society which fosters distrust and unhappiness by its non-observance of individuals' rights. We are all happier if we respect each other's autonomy, even when we think that the other person is mistaken.

BENEFICENCE—

Beneficence is the doing of good for another. It is usually accepted by health care professionals that we have a moral obligation to act for the best welfare of other persons. This is referred to as the *principle of beneficence*. This is a particularly important ethical

principle for health care professionals because our special education and training give us the capacity to help other persons in
ways in which they cannot help themselves. Specifically, through
our special skills as health care professionals, we have the ability
to help relieve the suffering caused by disease.

COMPETENCE—

Competence is really a legal term which refers to the patient's ability to exercise moral autonomy based upon one's ability to reason.
If reasoning is significantly impaired the patient is not able to exercise autonomy. In such cases, someone who is competent must be
chosen to make decisions on behalf of the patient. Whether a patient is competent or not is ultimately determined by the court,
but testimony by health professionals reflecting their evaluation of
the mental status of the patient should be important in making
such judgments.

CONSEQUENTIALIST ETHICS—

Consequentialist ethics are ethical theories which argue that the
moral rightness or wrongness of actions depends upon their outcome. Utilitarianism, advocated by John Stuart Mill, is a classic example of this kind of ethical theory. It argues that what makes an
action morally right (or wrong) is the happiness (or unhappiness)
it produces.

DEONTOLOGICAL ETHICS—

In contrast with consequentialist ethical theories, deontological
theories of ethics argue that the moral rightness or wrongness of
actions depends not upon their outcomes, but rather upon
whether or not the actions conform to the rules of ethics, i.e.,
whether or not they fulfill a moral duty. According to deontological theories, an action can be morally correct even if it causes
many people a great deal of suffering. One of the most well-
known deontological ethicists was Immanuel Kant, who argued
that all ethics could be derived from one fundamental principle,
which he called the "Categorical Imperative." This commands
that "One should act only upon those maxims that one would be
willing for everyone to act upon."

ETHICAL ABSOLUTISM—

Ethical absolutism is the opposite of ethical relativism. Absolutism holds that there are real moral values which hold true of all people at all times, whether they aware of those values or not.

ETHICAL RELATIVISM—

Ethical relativism is the theory that all moral values are relative to the society or culture. They are rules, peculiar to each society, governing interpersonal behavior. Many different cultures hold significantly different moral beliefs from us. According to ethical relativism, those beliefs are not wrong, they are just "different." Likewise, our beliefs may be "right" for us, but not necessarily right for any other social group.

JUSTICE—

In the health care context, two different sorts of justice frequently come into the decision-making process.

The first is *distributive justice*. Distributive justice has to do with the allocation of goods, in our context, with the allocation of scarce health care resources. Who should have a bed in the ICU? Who should receive the kidney transplant when not everyone who needs one can get one?

The second area of justice has to do with respecting the moral and legal rights of the individual. Justice requires that the physicians usually keep privileged patient information confidential. But in some cases, where the rights of innocent third parties are at risk, as with a tuberculosis or syphilis carrier, an interest in the public health can override the individual's right to confidentiality.

NON-MALEFICENCE—

Related to the principle of beneficence, the principle of non-maleficence requires that no harm be done to the patient. It may be familiar to the health care professional in the rule, *Primum non nocere* ("Above all, do no harm"). It is slightly different from the principle of beneficence in that it does not require that we actively help, but only that we not actively harm.

PATERNALISM—

Paternalism means to make decisions on someone else's behalf, just as a father makes decisions on behalf of his children. This may include going against what the individual involved says or wants on the presumption that we know better than the individual what is really in his or her best welfare.

Weak paternalism is defined as acting paternalistically towards someone who cannot make responsible choices for himself, for example a young child or an adult suffering from dementia. It is generally agreed that this can be morally proper since there is no autonomy that can be violated.

Strong paternalism, on the other hand means acting paternalistically towards someone who is mentally competent. Strong paternalism is morally controversial. Opinion runs generally, though by no means universally, against it.

SANCTITY OF LIFE—

An oft-mentioned principle of medical ethics, the sanctity of life, holds that all life, especially human life, is sacred. It is not within the domain of human purview to decide who or when one of us lives or dies.

The substance of the sanctity of life principle has been interpreted in various ways. Some have understood it to mean that all human life should be prolonged as long as humanly possible. Many people believe that the withholding of treatment from irreversibly and terminally ill patients is consistent with the sanctity of life when death is irrevocably imminent, i.e., when intervention would only prolong the dying process. On the other hand, many people, such as D.C. Thomasma, have extended the argument to conclude that the withholding or withdrawing of lifesaving treatment is consistent with the sanctity of life when the patient suffers an irreversible condition which renders the continuation of his or her life cruel rather than kind.

UTILITARIANISM—

Utilitarianism is an ethical theory formulated in England in the late 18th century by Jeremy Bentham. Its most famous proponent was John Stuart Mill. Utilitarianism, a consequentialist theory of ethics, holds that an action is morally right to the degree to which it contributes to the general happiness. If an action unnecessarily detracts from the general happiness by causing pain or suffering, it is morally wrong.

VIRTUE ETHICS—
Virtue ethicists argue that morality is really not found in either the consequences of actions or in the conformity of motives or actions with some moral law. Rather, morality has to do with character traits.

Thus the morally admirable person will be one who approaches the challenges of life with such virtues as courage, temperance, and generosity. The development of such character traits is perhaps more important than strict adherence to rules. It might also be the case that possession of the virtues may be a more reliable guide to morally correct actions than strict adherence to some moral law.

Brief Bibliography of Medical Ethics

Abrams N, and Brucker M (eds) *Medical Ethics: A Clinical Textbook and Reference for Health Care Professionals,* Cambridge, MA: MIT Press, 1983.
American College of Physicians, *Ethics Manual,* Philadelphia, PA: American College of Physicians, 1984.
  Originally published in *Annals of Internal Medicine* 101:129–37 and 263–74 (1984). It is now available as a pamphlet from the ACP. (Write to: Subscriber Service Division, American College of Physicians, 4200 Pine Street, Philadelphia, PA 19104.) Highly recommended.
Arras J, and Hunt R (eds.). *Ethical Issues in Modern Medicine,* Palo Alto, CA: Mayfield Publishing, 1983.
  This is an anthologized textbook containing articles on a wide range of ethical issues in medicine. Included are selections on the ethical complexion of the patient-provider relationship.
Beauchamp T, and Childress J. *Principles of Biomedical Ethics,* New York: Oxford University Press, 1983.
  One of the most widely used textbooks in medical ethics. Discusses many of the philosophical principles of ethics and shows how they may apply in medical contexts.
Mappes TA, and Zembaty JS (eds.). *Biomedical Ethics,* New York: McGraw-Hill, 1986.
  This anthologized text covers a variety of topics and includes around fifty pages on ethical decision making.

President's Commission for the Study of Ethical Issues in Medicine and in Biomedical and Behavioral Research.
    This Commission has published a number of seminal volumes. They offer sound advice. All are available from the US Government Printing Offices. The two volumes most relevant to our concerns are:
    1) *Making Health Care Decisions,* (vol.1) 1982.
    2) *Deciding to Forego Life-Sustaining Treatment,* 1983.
Rachels J. *The Elements of Moral Philosophy,* Philadelphia: Temple University Press, 1986.
    A useful general introduction to ethical principles and ethical reasoning. Not specifically on medical ethics.

Appendix I

The Living Will
and
Durable Power of
Attorney

The Living Will

What is a Living Will? It is a statement, signed by you and witnessed, which tells your family and your doctor your directions about life-prolonging medical procedures when your condition is hopeless and there is no chance of regaining what you consider to be a meaningful life.

●

Why do you need a Living Will? Medical advances can now keep you "alive" when your mind is gone and your body has stopped functioning naturally. Under constitutional and common law, you have the right to refuse treatment. A Living Will gives you the opportunity to express your wishes *in advance*, since you may not be able to make them known when it becomes important to do so.

●

What are "life-prolonging procedures"? These may include hooking you up to a machine when you cannot breathe on your own, performing operations or prescribing antibiotics that cannot realistically increase your chance of recovery, starting your heart mechanically when it has stopped beating, or feeding you by tube. You may, if you wish, specifically list on your Living Will the procedures you would or would *not* want administered. (If you do not include specifics, the general directions on the Declaration will stand for your wishes regarding treatment under the circumstances described. Your doctor and others will be informed that you want only comfort measures.)

●

What are comfort measures? Medication, nursing care and other treatment administered for the purpose of keeping you as comfortable and free from pain as possible.

●

The Living Will and durable power of attorney are reprinted with the permission of the Society for the Right to Die.

What is meant by "Other instructions/comments"?
Your Living Will should say exactly what *you* want it to say. This
means that you are free to add any directions to it that you wish.
Space is provided for this.

•

**Can you choose someone else to speak for you if you
cannot speak for yourself?** Your Living Will provides for this. It
offers you a second protection in allowing you to name a person
you trust (your "proxy") to make medical decisions for you in accordance with your wishes at a time when you cannot make them
for yourself.

•

Should your Living Will be witnessed? You should sign it
and date it in the presence of two witnesses. These may be any
adult persons of your choice.

•

What should you do with your Living Will? It is important that your family knows how you feel, and your Living Will
provides an opportunity to open up discussions of a subject that is
too often not talked about. You should give a copy of the signed
document to the people who might someday have to produce it
on your account. If you have a family doctor, it is most important
that you discuss it with him or her as well, and have a copy placed
in your medical file. If you do not have a family doctor, it is doubly
important that you discuss it with someone close to you. You
should also keep a copy among your important personal papers, in
a place known to your family, so it can be easily located. You
might also carry a card in your wallet stating that you have signed
a Living Will and indicating where it can be found. Do *not* place it
in a safety deposit box, where it would not be readily available
when needed. If you change doctors, make sure your new doctor
has a copy.

•

Is a Living Will legally binding? You have the constitutional and common-law right to refuse any treatment you do not want. Living Wills have been given weight in court decisions as evidence of a person's intent. Even though your state may not yet have passed a Living Will law, it is the best protection available to you until it does. In fact, a doctor or hospital treating you against your wishes (or those put forward by your proxy) may be liable for damages.

The laws of states that have passed Living Will legislation* contain the document form to be used by residents of those states. If you live in a state that has a Living Will law, you can obtain the appropriate form, along with instructions for its use, from the Society for the Right to Die. In addition, you may sign and give to your family and doctor the Society's Living Will. In that way you will be telling them your *personal* wishes. The Society's document can be especially important to you, too, if you are traveling and become hospitalized in a state without a Living Will law.

•

How can you make sure your Living Will will be viewed as an up-to-date document? Review it occasionally, and initial and date it, to show that it continues to express your choices accurately. You may make additions, changes, or deletions, provided they are clearly initialed and dated. Make sure any changes are shown on all copies, too. (You can, of course, revoke your Living Will at any time if you have a change of mind.)

•

Does a Living Will affect life insurance? No—and nearly all the Living Will laws that have been passed clearly state that new insurance applications cannot be turned down or existing policies affected by the signing of a Living Will. Signing a Living Will, or

---

*Alabama, Alaska, Arizona, Arkansas, California, Colorado, Connecticut, Delaware, Florida, Georgia, Hawaii, Idaho, Illinois, Indiana, Iowa, Kansas, Louisiana, Maine, Maryland, Mississippi, Missouri, Montana, Nevada, New Hampshire, New Mexico, North Carolina, Oklahoma, Oregon, South Carolina, Tennessee, Texas, Utah, Vermont, Virginia, Washington, West Virginia, Wisconsin, Wyoming, and the District of Columbia. (As of December 1987.)

Living Will Declaration

INSTRUCTIONS Consult this column for help and guidance.	To My Family, Doctors, and All Those Concerned with My Care
This declaration sets forth your directions regarding medical treatment.	I, _____, being of sound mind, make this statement as a directive to be followed if I become unable to participate in decisions regarding my medical care. If I should be in an incurable or irreversible mental or physical condition with no reasonable expectation of recovery, I direct my attending physician to withhold or withdraw treatment that merely prolongs my dying. I further direct that treatment be limited to measures to keep me comfortable and to relieve pain.
You have the right to refuse treatment you do not want, and you may request the care you do want.	These directions express my legal right to refuse treatment. Therefore I expect my family, doctors, and everyone concerned with my care to regard themselves as legally and morally bound to act in accord with my wishes, and in so doing to be free of any legal liability for having followed my directions.
You may list specific treatment you do *not* want. For example: **Cardiac resuscitation** **Mechanical respiration** **Artificial feeding/fluids** **by tubes**	I especially do not want: _____ _____ _____ _____

Otherwise, your general statement, top right, will stand for your wishes.

You may want to add instructions for care you *do* want—for example, pain medication; or that you prefer to die at home if possible.

Other instructions/comments:

_____

_____

_____

_____

If you want, you can name someone to see that your wishes are carried out, but you do not have to do this.

Proxy Designation Clause: Should I become unable to communicate my instructions as stated above, I designate the following person to act in my behalf:

Name _____

Address _____

If the person I have named above is unable to act in my behalf, I authorize the following person to do so:

Name _____

Address _____

Sign and date here in the presence of two adult witnesses, who should also sign.

Signed: _____   Date: _____

Witness: _____   Witness: _____

Keep the signed original with your personal papers at home. Give signed copies to your doctors, family, and to your proxy.

Review your Declaration from time to time; initial and date it to show it still expresses your intent.

terminating artificial life-prolonging treatment, or not starting treatment at all, is *not* considered suicide or assisted suicide.

●

How did the Living Will originate? The term "Living Will" has become part of our everyday vocabulary, and yet few are aware of its history. In 1967, a Chicago attorney, Luis Kutner, addressed a Society meeting. By law, he said, a patient cannot be subjected to treatment against his or her wishes. When the patient's condition is such that neither consent nor refusal can be expressed, a physician might assume that everything possible must be done to preserve life. To prevent treatment that may be contrary to the patient's will, Mr. Kutner proposed that a person while still of sound mind draw up a document as a "testament permitting death."

At that meeting in 1967, Society members were asked to "draw up such a Living Will which might serve as a sample or a suggestion" for others. Since then, there have been several versions of the Living Will and millions of copies distributed.

Durable Power of Attorney

Hopelessly ill patients often lose their capacity to make decisions about medical treatment. Advanced directives—commonly called Living Wills—are an important means of preserving their right to refuse artificial, life-sustaining "heroic" measures that can only prolong dying.

A second form of protection of the patient's right of self-determination is offered by the appointment of someone to make health-care decisions on behalf of the appointer if incapacitated—that is, an agent as authorized by a proxy provision in a "Living Will" statute or by a "durable power of attorney" statute.

What is a durable power of attorney?

An ordinary power of attorney is a means of authorizing another person to make decisions and take actions on your behalf—for example, to pay your bills, from your bank account if you are on an extended trip or in a hospital. This authority lapses if you, the "principal," become incompetent.

A durable power of attorney, however, is an authorization that remains (or, in some states, becomes) effective after the principal has become incompetent. All 50 states now have statutes legally recognizing and defining durable powers of attorney.

Traditionally and historically, powers of attorney, whether ordinary or durable, have been used in connection with actions affecting the principal's property. According to the authors of a comprehensive study on the subject, there is nothing in any statute or court decision that restricts the use of this authorization to matters of property alone; they believe that "any power of attorney, whether ordinary or durable, can be used for any purpose that is not contrary to law or public policy of a given state."* The durable power of attorney, therefore, offers a potentially useful legal instrument by which you can protect your right to refuse life-sustaining procedures in the event of a hopeless condition and incapacity to make decisions.

What do durable power statutes provide?

There is no single, clear-cut answer to this question, for the statutes vary from state to state. Some states authorize a durable power that becomes effective immediately and continues after the appointing principal has become incompetent, while in other states the power becomes effective only after the principal has become incompetent. Some impose specific restrictions on its use. Some require particular language to be used and some have special witnessing and filing requirements. In view of these variations, as well as of the significance of empowering another to make health-care decisions for you, it is important to seek the advice and assistance of an attorney in your state to draw up a durable power of attorney form.

Five durable power of attorney statutes address the issue of medical treatment decisions. Two of them—California's and Rhode Island's—specifically authorize decisions to withhold or

---

*Francis J. Collin, Jr., John J. Lombard, Jr.,Albert L. Moses, Harley J. Spitler, Drafting the Durable Power of Attorney, R.P.W. Publishing Corp., Lexington, SC (1984), p. 21.

withdraw life support. (Durable Power of Attorney for Health Care forms for both California and Rhode Island are available from the Society for the Right to Die.) The durable power statutes of Colorado, North Carolina and Pennsylvania (and a related statute in Maryland) authorize attorneys-in-fact to consent to medical treatment but are silent about whether they can refuse it. Finally, four other states have indicated that a durable power of attorney can be used to terminate treatment: through opinions of their courts (Arizona and New Jersey), of the state attorney general (New York), and of a district attorney (Nevada).

What is a proxy?

Another method of appointing someone to make medical decisions on your behalf if you are unable to do so is by appointing a "proxy" in your Living Will. Seven of the Living Will statutes—Delaware, Florida, Louisiana, Texas, Utah, Virginia, and Wyoming—specifically authorize the appointment of a health-care proxy to refuse life-sustaining treatment. In addition, the Living Will statutes of four other states—Hawaii, Idaho, Indiana, and Iowa—indirectly authorize such appointments.

How do attorneys-in-fact with durable power compare with proxies?

Both are designed to make health-care decisions on your behalf. States vary as to which is the more legally viable route. In some states, the proxy is more explicitly endorsed (e.g., Virginia) while in others, the durable power is more clearly protected (e.g. California). To ensure maximum protection, you should appoint the same person as attorney-in-fact and proxy. Once again, we suggest you consult a local attorney about your state's laws for appointing an agent to make health-care decisions.

Why should you appoint an agent?

The clinical circumstances of a future illness and available treatment options are unpredictable. For this reason, it can be a significant protection to designate in advance an agent empowered to make decisions on your behalf that are based both on personal knowledge of your own wishes and direct consultation with your physician.

You may wish to make use of the durable power of attorney, authorizing decision making in any or all of the following areas:

1. To give or withhold consent to specific medical or surgical measures with reference to the principal's condition, prognosis, and known wishes regarding terminal care; to authorize appropriate end-of-life care, including pain-relieving procedures.
2. To grant releases to medical personnel.
3. To employ and discharge medical personnel.
4. To have access to and to disclose medical records and other personal information.
5. To resort to court, if necessary, to obtain court authorization regarding medical treatment decisions.
6. To expend (or withhold) funds necessary to carry out medical treatment.

Whom should you appoint?

The person you appoint could be your spouse, a relative, or a close friend. Above all, it should be someone you trust and have confidence in—someone who is familiar with your own feelings about terminal care, who supports them, and who would be likely to make the same decisions you would make if you were able to do so. You should also make sure that you choose someone who is willing to take action on your behalf, who does not shrink from the burden of what may be a difficult and painful responsibility. All of this will require careful thought on your part and full consultation with your agent of choice.

You should also consider appointing more than one agent, the second to act in the event that the first is unavailable when needed.

Appendix II

Formulating the Limited Treatment Plan

The process of developing a limited treatment plan is neither simple nor emotionally easy. This is true for all parties that might be involved—patient, family, physician, and other members of the health care team. To assist in that difficult process, this appendix provides some suggestions under the headings "When," "Where," "Who," "What," and "How." It concludes with a sample chart designed for bedside or patient file use to notify health care providers of the patient's limited treatment plan.

When

Appropriate times for discussion of a limited treatment plan include:

1) Shortly after the diagnosis of a debilitating or life-threatening illness. This should not be done on the same occasion as informing the patient of the diagnosis. Rather, a follow-up conference should be arranged, allowing the patient time to recover from the emotional shock of diagnosis.

2) Prior to potentially life-threatening intervention, such as major surgery.

3) Around the time of a major clinical milestone. This could be either deterioration pertaining to a long-standing illness (such as kidney failure) or the appearance of clinical signs of irremediable illness (such as recurrent metastases).

4) The patient (or family) requests a meeting.

5) When illness prompts consideration of a change of treatment settings, such as transfer from the nursing home to the hospital.

6) A major event in the life of the care giver, either the care giver at home or the physician.

7) A financial change of status, such as the patient running out of private funds.

Where

There are three likely places for the limited treatment conference.

1) The office—Try to schedule this so that ample time is available, such as at the end of the day when there are no other pressing engagements.

2) The hospital—Arrange for a conference room or use of a private patient room to maximize privacy.

3) The home.

Who

This will vary, depending upon both the nature of the illness and the location of the conference. For example, a discharge planner might be important in the hospital setting, while a home care specialist might be important in the office or home setting. The number of persons involved in the actual planning conference with the patient (or appropriate decision maker) should be kept to a minimum in order to avoid intimidating the patient. This means, however, that many individuals who play an important role, such as nutritionists, physical therapists, and so on must be consulted closely both before and after the actual conference.

What

Developing a limited treatment plan is not simply a medical matter. A number of things in addition to the medical facts must be brought out into the open. Discussion should cover:

1) The patient's medical history, present condition, and prognosis.
2) Given the patient's condition and prognosis, the various possible treatment options must be identified.
3) The patient's financial status must be reviewed. Private monies must be determined and third party coverage evaluated.
4) Of the various treatment options identified, which are financially feasible?
5) Of the various treatment options identified, which are practical and available? (e.g., is there a nursing home bed available? Can the family manage the proposed treatment at home practically?)
6) What are the patient's values? (If the patient is incompetent, seek guidance from advance directives or from family members concerning patient's previously expressed values.)
7) Given the options which are feasible, which best suits the patient's values? (This decision must be made ultimately by the patient or the designated decision maker.)

How

1) The professional staff should review the team's goals and recommendations prior to the conference. An agenda or discussion "flow sheet" should be prepared.

2) If appropriate, legal advice should be obtained beforehand.
3) The conference discussion should begin with a brief, business-like chronology of the events leading up to the conference.
4) The conference should formally establish who is the appropriate decision maker. This is especially important if the patient is not the decision maker.
5) The conference should then follow the prepared agenda.
6) Keep the information in a business-like tone. The meeting will be emotionally charged, and if the plan is to be thoughtfully developed the meeting must proceed in a calm manner. Keep in mind that the family is preparing for death in a manner similar to the patient.
7) End the meeting with a clear outline of the decisions made. If any decisions remain unresolved, leave the patient with the choices and a deadline for making them or schedule a follow-up meeting before concluding the conference.
8) The physician is responsible for entering a progress note in the patient's record indicating:
   1. date and time of the meeting and the note
   2. a list of who attended
   3. a list of the decisions made
   4. identity of the authoritative decision maker
9) Finally, the physician should update the limited treatment chart posted in the patient's record.

Sample Limited Treatment Chart
LIMITED TREATMENT PLAN

Name: _____ Date: ___/___/___

Medical Ident. No: _____ Rm No:_____

Diagnostic Plan:
  Invasive testing:
  No   Yes
  ☐   ☐   Hospital transfer/admission: _____
  ☐   ☐   Endoscopy: _____
  ☐   ☐   Tissue Biopsy/surgery: _____
  Non-invasive testing:
  No   Yes
  ☐   ☐   Hospital transfer/admission: _____
  ☐   ☐   Radiology: _____
  ☐   ☐   Venopuncture: _____
Treatment Plan:
  Hospitalization:
  No   Yes
  ☐   ☐   Clinical deterioration: _____
  ☐   ☐   Emergency surgery: _____
  ☐   ☐   Intensive care: _____
  ☐   ☐   Specialty palliative care: _____
  Resuscitation:
  No   Yes
  ☐   ☐   Basic life support: _____
  ☐   ☐   Electro-chemical code (prolonged): _____
  ☐   ☐   Intubation and mechanical vent: _____
  ☐   ☐   Invasive cardiac support: _____
  Medications:
  No   Yes
  ☐   ☐   Chemotherapy: _____
  ☐   ☐   Antibiotics: _____
  ☐   ☐   Other: _____
  Nutrition-Hydration:
  No   Yes
  ☐   ☐   Spoon-feeding: _____
  ☐   ☐   Nasogastric tube feeding: _____
  ☐   ☐   Gastrostomy tube: _____
  ☐   ☐   Limited IVs (3 days): _____
Personal designee for decisions:_____
Address:_____
Phone: _____ Rel: _____
Others to be notified in case of clinical change:_____

INDEX

A

Abandonment, 118, 124, 216
  and euthanasia, 165
Abuse
  elder, 58, 199
  in research, 88
Administration
  in long-term care settings,
    187–88
Advance directives, 38–39, 238
  on euthanasia, 166
  on nutritional supports, 139
  on treatment procedures,
    102–03, 111, 118, 127
  and ventilators, 113
  See also Legal issues, Living
    Wills, Resuscitation
Advocacy, 16–17, 71
  and allocation, 121, 217
  and research, 95–96
AIDS, 186
Allocation issues, 121, 124
  See also Financial issues
Alzheimer's disease, 22, 35
  and human research, 89, 91,
    93
American Association of
  Retired Persons, 219
American College of Physicians,
  122
  on resuscitation, 145
American Hemlock Society, 157
American Medical Association
  on euthanasia, 162
  on nutritional support, 138
  on resuscitation, 145, 148

on treatment, 117, 119
Amputation, 130
Aristotle
  on self-rule, 25
Arthritis, 104
Attorneys-in-fact, 240
  See also Legal issues
Autonomy, 9
  and CPR, 145–46
  defined, 6, 25–26, 225
  and diagnostic intervention,
    111
  funeral planning, 220
  at home, 196–97
  incompetency and, 22, 37–
    39, 88, 120
  and limiting treatment, 123–
    25
  in long-term care facility,
    189–90
  and nutritional supports, 134,
    138–39, 141
  preserving, 15, 44–45
  See also Paternalism

B

The Belmont Report, 87–88
Beneficence, 5–6
  and CPR, 149
  defined, 225–26
  and euthanasia, 162–63
  incompetency and, 38, 120
  and research, 88
Bereavement, 104
Biopsies, 106–07, 156
Blood sampling, 106